Choosing a Model

Caring for Patients with Cardiovascular and Respiratory

USING NURSING MODELS SERIES

General Editors:

Jane E Schober SRN, RCNT, DipN Ed, DipN (Lond), RNT
Lecturer, Nursing Studies, Institute of Advanced Nursing Education,
Royal College of Nursing

Christine Webb BA, MSc, PhD, SRN, RSCN, RNT
Principal Lecturer in Nursing, Department of Nursing, Health and
Applied Social Studies, Bristol Polytechnic, Bristol

The views expressed in this book are those of the authors of individual chapters
and do not necessarily reflect the opinions of the series editors.

Other titles in the Series:

Elderly Care: Towards Holistic Nursing
Edited by Jane Easterbrook

Mental Handicap: Facilitating Holistic Care
Edited by Paul Barber

Psychiatric Nursing: Person to Person
Edited by Blair Collister

Women's Health: Midwifery and Gynaecological Nursing
Edited by Christine Webb

Choosing a Model

Caring for Patients with Cardiovascular and Respiratory Problems

Helen Chalmers
BA, SRN, RNT, DipN (LOND)

Senior Tutor, Continuing Education Department,
Bath District Health Authority

Edward Arnold

A division of Hodder & Stoughton
LONDON   BALTIMORE   MELBOURNE   AUCKLAND

© 1988 Helen Chalmers

First published in Great Britain 1988

British Library Cataloguing in Publication Data

Choosing a model: caring for patients with
   cardiovascular and respiratory problems.
   1. Cardiovascular patient. Nursing 2.
   Respiratory patient. Nursing
   I. Chalmers, Helen   II. Series
   610.73'691

   ISBN 0-340-41776-5

Typeset in Linotron Ehrhardt by Wearside Tradespools, Fulwell, Sunderland
Printed and bound in Great Britain for Edward Arnold, the educational,
academic and medical publishing division of Hodder & Stoughton Limited,
41 Bedford Square, London WC1B 3DQ at The Bath Press, Avon

Contents

List of Contributors

Helen Ashton SRN, DIPN (LOND), FETC was, until recently, a school nurse with Bath District Health Authority. She is currently working in the Continuing Education Department of the same Health Authority.

Helen Chalmers BA, SRN, RNT, DIPN (LOND) is a senior nurse tutor in the Continuing Education Department, Bath District Health Authority. She is course director in Bath to the London University Diploma in Nursing Course.

Anne Chew SRN, DIPN (LOND) was, until recently, a staff nurse on night duty at a community hospital in the Bath District Health Authority.

Vivien Crouch SRN, DIPN (LOND) works as a school nurse with Bath District Health Authority.

Margaret Doman SRN, RSCN, ONC, DIPN (LOND) worked as a staff nurse in the Paediatric Unit at the Royal United Hospital, Bath until 1987. She is currently a ward sister in the Paediatric Unit at Musgrove Park Hospital, Taunton.

Sarah Gunningham SRN, DIPN (LOND) works as a staff nurse on the Intensive Therapy Unit at Bristol Royal Infirmary.

Kate Harris SRN, HV CERT, DIPN (LOND) is a health visitor with Bath District Health Authority.

Timothy Holt SRN, DIPN (LOND) is a charge nurse on a mixed medical ward at the Royal United Hospital, Bath.

Marie May SRN, DIPN (LOND) works as a night sister in a community hospital in the Bath District Health Authority.

Valerie Newton SRN, DipN (LOND) worked, until recently, as a staff nurse on the Intensive Care Unit, Royal United Hospital, Bath and then completed the cardiothoracic course (ENB 249) at the Brompton Hospital, London. She is currently working in the Wellington Hospital, New Zealand.

Anne PM Williams SRN, DIPN (LOND) was, until recently, a ward sister in a community hospital in the Bath District Health Authority. Currently she works as a community nurse and is planning to train as a district nurse.

Preface

This book has been written with one aim in mind – to share with others the practical experiences gained by qualified nurses working in a variety of settings.

The common theme is that each chapter attempts to explore the usefulness of a particular model of nursing.

The contributors do not profess to be recognised authors within the field of nursing. Indeed, for many the compilation of a chapter seemed a daunting task. However, what they bring to this book is a commitment to take on the new challenges within nursing that face us all. Where they may differ from many who hopefully will read and be encouraged by this book, is in their shared experience of studying for the University of London Diploma in Nursing (new syllabus).

If just some of their enthusiasm for and commitment to enhancing the quality of care comes through to the readers of this book, then their hard work will be justified. If others are stimulated to take up the challenge that nursing models present, their hard work will be rewarded.

Helen Chalmers
Bath, 1988

N.B. Personal details have been altered to maintain the anonymity of all patients featured in this book.

Acknowledgements

I should like to thank all those who have contributed chapters to this book both for their initial enthusiasm and for their hard work in turning that enthusiasm into the written word. I acknowledge too their patience in waiting for the whole project to come to fruition.

My thanks go also to Christine Webb for offering me the opportunity to edit this book and for continued encouragement as the work progressed.

I owe an enormous debt of gratitude to Jayne Everett without whose time and skill on the word processor there might never have been a book at all!

I

Introduction: Choice

Helen Chalmers

There appears to be a continuing and mounting emphasis within health care on standard setting (e.g., RCN, 1980, 1981; Kitson, 1987), quality assurance (e.g., Donabedian, 1966, 1969; Maxwell, 1984; Kitson, 1986) and accountability, (e.g., Bergman, 1981; Crow, 1983; UKCC, 1984). In part this reflects the move towards greater cost effectiveness that characterised the management restructuring of the National Health Service in 1984. In addition many health carers wish to offer a quality of care that both they and the public find acceptable and that can be achieved within the current financial climate.

Bergman (1981) has cited a better informed public as one of the societal reasons why nursing has become preoccupied with accountability. More information generally leads to an awareness that situations can be responded to in a number of different ways. It becomes clear that decisions may need to be taken and choices made. There is a certain ambiguity for a health service which is financially constrained at a time when many people require it to have the capability of responding to their needs in a flexible and sensitive way.

Against a background of change therefore, nurses are trying to improve standards of care and are involved in making choices themselves and in providing a range of choices to patients and clients. Much has already been written about the nature and importance of informed consent (RCN, 1977; Faulder, 1985; Melia, 1986; Pyne, 1986; Wells, 1986). Perhaps the time is now right for a fuller consideration of the issue of informed choice.

The nursing process and choice

The introduction of the nursing process was not the overwhelming success that many nurses had hoped for. There were a number of reasons for this and one was certainly its uncritical acceptance by some nurses. Coupled with this was the way in which its adoption as a means of planning and delivering nursing care was imposed by those who held most power in the nursing world (for example GNC, 1977). The *Report of the Nursing Process Evaluation Working Group* (Hayward, 1986: p. 7) has recently described such a move as 'well-intentioned, somewhat premature'.

Added to this was the concern of many nurses, that, alone, the nursing process offered nothing new and was failing to improve standards of care. Nevertheless, there were other nurses who claimed that the nursing process was significantly improving standards in many areas.

How was it possible for two such opposing views to be current at the same time? A plausible solution can be put forward by considering what else was uppermost in the minds of nurses when the nursing process was introduced. At that time there was a move away from traditional task-orientated approaches to nursing care. Many nurses saw the emphasis on the individual as an integral part of the nursing process itself.

For these nurses *two* changes took place in their practice. First, they tried to reorientate the care they offered such that individuals were of central importance. Second, they adopted the problem-solving approach called the nursing process. It is difficult to evaluate the relative contributions of these two changes in any improvements in standards of care.

Yet other nurses were attempting to implement the nursing process but found it could be a means of perpetuating task-orientated care. Thus Nurse X could be allocated the task of assessing all the new admissions while Nurse Y carried out various interventions. Nurse Y therefore might complete dressings and perhaps give out medicines. Meanwhile Nurse Z might spend time evaluating the care given by ensuring that tasks were completed and would be likely to write to this effect in the nursing records.

It was therefore not surprising that nurses became confused, perhaps even divided, about what the nursing process really was and how it provided the potential to improve standards of care. For many came the realisation that the nursing process, used in isolation, is an empty tool. It encourages nurses to assess patients but fails to offer guidance about the choices that must be made about assessment (Aggleton and Chalmers, 1986). For example, what information should be sought and recorded and what can be safely ignored? How might assessment be carried out most sensitively and effectively?

Similarly the nursing process advocates planned care but does not offer information on the way plans should be made or the nature of the goals that might be set. It further suggests that once goals are identified nurses should act to facilitate goal achievement, but there is no recognition that choices need to be made, that nurses might need guidance in deciding how best and when to intervene. Evaluation is commended as an essential fourth step of the nursing process but the ways in which this might be carried out are ignored.

There are, then, within the nursing process many choices to be made. Here are some questions that nurses might ask themselves – there are many others:

1 How should assessment be carried out?

2 What data should be gathered and what can be safely left on one side?
3 What type of goal-setting will most benefit the patient?
4 How can a choice be made between acting in this way or acting in that way?
5 How can the success, or otherwise, of nursing intervention be measured?

Such important choices need to be informed and nursing models offer one way in which this can happen. The nursing process is not a model of nursing but the nature of its steps – namely assessment, planning, intervention and evaluation – may be incorporated within a model. It is likely that those nurses who attempted to use the nursing process, but found it offered nothing new, were being guided not by the understandings of a nursing model but by traditional, usually medical, approaches to care.

Nursing models and choice

At present there does not exist sufficient nursing research conclusively to confirm or deny that nursing models make a significant contribution to standards of care. This is not, however, a reason for either ignoring their existence or resisting the opportunity to explore their possible value.

If nurses are to be accountable for their practice, they must address the issue of nursing models and the potential they provide for the establishment of a knowledge base from which informed choices can be made. It is no longer acceptable to deny the existence of nursing models or to plead ignorance of what they mean. If a nurse chooses *not* to work with a recognised nursing model, that decision must be justifiable and based on sound and up-to-date knowledge. The choice *not* to do something is as important as the choice *to* do something.

It was argued above that, in order to use the problem-solving approach to care called the nursing process, nurses have to make choices, for example about what or how to assess. However, nurses who do not claim to use a nursing model still gather data about people. On what do they base their decisions about the 'what' and 'how' of assessment? It was suggested that such choices might stem from the understandings associated with the medical model. It is also probable that nurses use ideas about what information is important and what is not, which they have developed as a result of nursing experience and past learning.

Such a 'private image' (McFarlane, 1986) of nursing is not to be undervalued, built as it is on experience within the field of nursing. However, were such nurses to be asked to make public their private image, this might pose some difficulties. Nevertheless, this is what the writers of nursing models have tried to do. They have put before the nursing profession at large, their considered views about the nature of nursing and in most instances they have attempted to analyse and support the elements within their models. By so doing they have laid themselves open to the kind of scrutiny and criticism that most practising nurses never experience.

Thus nurses are faced with a variety of nursing models on which care can be based and choices have to be made between one model and another. It is important that all models have something to say about the nature of people as this should enable a tentative choice to be made. Models are not describing a separate breed, called patients, but are attempting to identify commonalities between people and the way they live in a social world. Initially then it may be useful to consider whether or not the model conceptualises people in a way with which the nurse can identify.

An early opinion about a particular model might be formed by considering whether the model views people as a collection of behavioural subsystems (Johnson, 1980), as a self-care agent (Orem, 1980) or as a giver of meaning to situations (Riehl, 1980). Most nursing models will acknowledge the bio-psychosocial nature of people but will vary in the relative emphasis given to each aspect.

Whilst a start may be made on evaluating the apparent acceptability of a model by comparing the understandings it sets out about people with the beliefs held by the nurse, the choice of model must reflect a concern for the needs of patients.

Although it might be possible for the choice of model to be made for each individual patient, this is probably unnecessary and unrealistic. It would be inappropriate to take the notion of individuality too far. Each individual has a unique make-up but people share much in common. It is therefore likely that a chosen model can be used in a particular unit or department for the majority of people cared for there.

In a health district, then, there may be three or four models in current use in different areas. Each model might offer something special to the people requiring nursing care in those areas. Such a situation would be preferable to the imposition of one model of nursing in a given health district or to the haphazard and uncritical use of numerous models at the whim of any practising nurse.

It is essential that the choice of nursing model is made with care and that those making such choices realise the importance of the decision they are taking. A number of authors have attempted to provide guidelines for nurses in order to facilitate this process. (See for example, Riehl and Roy, 1980; Chinn and Jacobs, 1983; Meleis, 1985; Stanton, 1985.)

The choice of nursing model is not neutral and to select one particular model is to accept the major concepts contained within the model and the role of the nurse that it advocates. To choose, for example, Henderson's model (Henderson, 1966) is to recognise the ambiguity that exists between the notion of a nurse as an independent practitioner with a 'unique function' and the notion of a nurse who must act as a physician's assistant. To work with Orem's self-care model (Orem, 1980) highlights the importance of adults taking responsibility for their own health and that of their dependants.

However, selecting a nursing model by carefully considering the concepts contained within it can only be a beginning. What is also needed is for practising nurses to take up the challenges offered by models and to use them as a basis for planning and delivering care in a variety of clinical settings. Evaluation of the care that then takes place can help to inform subsequent choices.

It is the realisation that such experiences need to be shared as widely as possible with other practising nurses that has led to the contributors of this book writing about the use of specific nursing models in their clinical areas.

Models, theory and practice

The debate about the relationship between nursing theory and nursing practice is not new but seems to have been further highlighted by the development of nursing models. Nursing models cannot be considered as theories of nursing but may well lead to the development of theory at a later date and after repeated evaluations in a variety of nursing situations. Some nurses may argue that nursing models are only useful at an academic level and have little relevance to practice. This is to deny the crucial interdependence of models, theory and practice.

Some of the criticisms of nursing models have centred on the terminology that they use (e.g., Johnson, 1986). Certainly complicated language has little virtue *per se*, but unfamiliar and difficult words alone are not sufficient reason to discount the nursing model from which they come. If after careful consideration little of value is found within a model, *then* a decision might be taken to select a different conceptual framework. Traditionally nurses have worked with the medical model, the terminology of which only seems familiar through experience of its use.

Furthermore, those nurses who are searching for a simple model around which to plan and deliver care must carefully reflect on their understanding of the nature of people. If people were uncomplicated then a simple model might be appropriate, but the desire of many nurses to offer individuality of care centres on an acknowledgement of the complexity of human nature.

So, whilst accepting that many nursing models are of necessity complex, do they only offer a focus for theoretical, academic study or do they have the potential to inform nursing practice in such a way that standards of care might be enhanced?

To separate potential nursing theory from practice is impossible and to attempt it is unwise because their interdependence should be at the heart of any planned change in nursing. If initially, as would seem reasonable, models are carefully thought about, evaluated and discussed by groups of interested nurses, such apparently academic study is likely to affect subsequent practice. To explore the essence of a nursing model and to think through how it might work in practice, is to question existing methods of working and to consider alternative ways of planning and delivering care.

If such considerations lead to the use of a particular model in practice, yet more questioning and evaluating should take place which may well send nurses back to the published work of other nurses and health carers to further inform the care they offer.

Nursing models may be viewed as frameworks that indicate how care might be managed under ideal circumstances. Often such ideals are based on theoretical understandings which challenge traditional routines and procedures. However, without some notion of how care *might* be managed in different ways, there might be complacency about current standards. Reality shock has been described (Kramer, 1974) when learner nurses experience a discrepancy between care advocated in schools of nursing and care possible in clinical settings. A similar experience may confront nurses who recognise the potential of a nursing model but find it difficult to implement in practice.

The solution is not to recoil from sharing and discussing theoretical ideals but to help nurses make choices that are informed and can therefore be justified to others. This may go some way towards facilitating the management of change.

Theory and practice are inextricably intertwined. A knowledge of theory must inform practice and practice must be evaluated to validate theory. Nursing models are the early stages of nursing theory and as such should be rigorously debated by practising nurses. The care plans that follow are a modest attempt to stimulate and contribute to such debate.

References

Aggleton P & Chalmers H 1986 *Nursing Models and the Nursing Process.* Macmillan, London.
Bergman R 1981 Accountability: definitions and dimensions. *International Nursing Review*, **28**, 2: 53–59.
Chinn PL & Jacobs MK 1983 *Theory and Nursing.* CV Mosby, St Louis.
Crow R 1983 Professional responsibility! *Nursing Times*, **79**, 1: 19.

Donabedian A 1966 Evaluating the quality of medical care. *Millbank Memorial Fund Quarterly*, **44**, 3: 166–206.

Donabedian A 1969 Some issues in evaluating the quality of nursing care. *American Journal of Public Health*, **59**, 10: 1833–1836.

Faulder C 1985 *Whose body is it?* Virago Press, London.

General Nursing Council for England and Wales 1977 *A Statement of Educational Policy.* Circular 77/19/A.

Hayward J (Ed) 1986 *Report of the Nursing Process Evaluation Working Group.* Number 5. DHSS.

Henderson V 1966 *The Nature of Nursing.* Macmillan, New York.

Johnson D 1980 The behavioural system model for nursing. In *Conceptual Models for Nursing Practice*, JP Riehl & C Roy (Eds). Appleton-Century-Crofts, Norwalk.

Johnson M 1986 Model of perfection? *Nursing Times*, **82**, 42: 44.

Kitson AL 1986 The methods of measuring quality. *Nursing Times*, **82**: 32–34.

Kitson AL 1987 Raising standards of clinical practice – the fundamental issue of effective nursing practice. *Journal of Advanced Nursing*, **12**, 3: 321–329.

Kramer M 1974 *Reality Shock: Why Nurses Leave Nursing!* CV Mosby, London.

Maxwell R 1984 Quality assessment in health. *British Medical Journal*, **288**: 1470–1472.

McFarlane J 1986 The Value of Models for Care. In *Models for Nursing*, B Kershaw & J Salvage (Eds). John Wiley, Chichester.

Meleis AI 1985 *Theoretical Nursing: Development and Progress.* Lippincott, Philadelphia.

Melia K 1986 Dangerous territory. *Nursing Times*, **82**, 21: 27.

Orem DE 1980 *Nursing: Concepts of Practice.* McGraw-Hill, New York.

Pyne R 1986 Tell me honestly. *Nursing Times*, **82**, 21: 25–26.

Riehl JP 1980 The Riehl Interaction Model. In *Conceptual Models for Nursing Practice*, JP Riehl & C Roy (Eds). Appleton-Century-Crofts, Norwalk.

Riehl JP & Roy C (Eds) 1980 *Conceptual Models for Nursing Practice.* Appleton-Century-Crofts, Norwalk.

Royal College of Nursing 1977 *Ethics Related to Research in Nursing.* RCN, London.

Royal College of Nursing 1980 *Standards of Nursing Care.* RCN, London.

Royal College of Nursing 1981 *Towards Standards.* RCN, London.

Stanton M 1985 Nursing theories and the nursing process. In *Nursing Theories*, JB George (Ed). Prentice-Hall, London.

UKCC 1984 *Code of Professional Conduct*, 2nd Ed. UKCC, London.

Wells R 1986 The great conspiracy. *Nursing Times*, **82**, 21: 22–25.

2

Care plan for a girl with asthma, using Roy's Adaptation model

Helen Ashton and Vivien Crouch

Introduction

According to Price (1984), asthma appears to be one of the most common causes of ill health in childhood. The Court Report (1976) and Anderson *et al.* (1981) indicate that children with asthma have frequent absences from school which has implications for their social, psychological and educational development. This care plan illustrates the nursing care and support offered by a school nurse to a 17-year-old school girl with chronic asthma attending a large single sex comprehensive school. The Roy Adaptation model of nursing provided the framework for gathering information, identifying problems and indicating where intervention should be concentrated.

Review of current literature

Scadding (1983) points to the lack of agreement over what is meant by the term 'asthma' but offers a primary definition:

asthma is a disease characterised by wide variations over short periods of time in resistence to flow in intrapulmonary airways.

There appear to be differing views in the classification of categories of asthma in the literature such as the use of the terms 'extrinsic' and 'intrinsic' asthma. Gregg (1983) argues that such terms can lead to confusion and may be better avoided. Therefore Levy and Bell's (1984) definition

appears appropriate when defining asthma in childhood:

(a) variable airways obstruction as shown by a history of recurrent wheeze, shortness of breath or cough and a subsequent response to anti-asthmatic treatment or (b) variation in peak expiratory flow rates of 20 per cent or more, or both (a) and (b).

Initially this appears to be an involved definition but Anderson *et al.* (1981) argue that children with recurrent wheezing illness with an underlying disease process essentially similar to that of asthma may not receive appropriate drug therapy. Similarly Lee *et al.* (1983) and Levy and Bell (1984) argue that asthma may remain undiagnosed because the symptoms may be limited to such signs as wheezing after exercise or recurrent cough. Thus a definition of asthma embracing the variety of physical symptoms that children may experience might lead to different treatment strategies. Speight *et al.* (1983) suggest that prophylactic drug therapy for asthma in such children appears to improve their health and reduce absence from school.

According to Colver (1984) the detection of children with asthma, the instigation or improvement of treatment and dissemination of information about childhood asthma to families and teachers may improve the health and therefore school attendance of most children with asthma. Colver argues that if teachers are informed about the importance of certain aspects of management of asthma, they are more likely to let children keep their inhalers with them in school and are less likely to send home a child who is wheezing.

Nash *et al.* (1985) suggest the school nurse may be the person most concerned with maintaining contact with teachers about the relevant health problems of the individual child. Newby and Nicoll (1985) point to the advantage of early identification of health problems (such as untreated asthma) which appear to impede a child's educational, psychological and social progress at school. Mead (1982) argues that the school nurse may be in the best position to recognise undiagnosed asthma. An awareness that not all children with asthma present with wheezing may lead the nurse to suspect that a child with other symptoms, for example shortness of breath after exercise or an unwillingness to take part in sport, may have asthma.

Once asthma is diagnosed, Lewis and Lewis' (1984) view is that children should be given sufficient medical treatment to enable a normal life to be led and should be encouraged to take part in sports, especially swimming. They argue that exercise-induced asthma can be controlled by sodium cromoglycate (Intal) or beta$_2$ sympathomimetic drugs (for example salbutamol) before exercise. However Lewis and Lewis also state that cross country running is not suitable for most asthmatic children. In addition Mead (1982) argues that by providing children and their parents with adequate information about asthma, asthmatic attacks may be minimised. According to Mead adequate instruction in the use of prophylactic measures and their benefits should be given and regularly reinforced.

Nash *et al.* (1985) point to the importance of properly managed exercise which may strengthen resistance to asthmatic attacks. Furthermore, Mead (1982) argues that such exercise may alter a child's view of asthma from it being an incapacitating illness to something which can be managed, thereby allowing a child to take part in a full range of school activities. Similarly Busfield's (1982) view is that programmes of physical activity may help children with asthma by enhancing their tolerance of exercise and by increasing their self-confidence and social and psychological independence.

The literature explored so far demonstrates not only the traditional physiological view of asthma and its management, but also begins to identify the social and psychological implications of living with a medical diagnosis of asthma. Furthermore, children with asthma may have anxieties which have their origin in both the physiological manifestations of asthma and in other sources as well. The more psychological aspects of coping with asthma are to be found in the literature. For example Cohen and Lask (1983) point to the relationship between emotional disturbance and the onset of asthma attacks in individuals whose 'bronchi are constitutionally hyper-reactive' and 'predispose' them 'to develop the disorder'. Cohen and Lask also point to the role that family stress may have in exacerbating a child's asthmatic symptoms. Price (1985) offers strategies which may help such tensions; for example, the provision of information about asthma to the family may enhance the parents' understanding so that a more appropriate response is made to the child's future asthmatic attacks.

Justification for choice of nursing model

The Roy Adaptation model was chosen as a basis for this care plan because it uses an approach which focuses on individuals who are having difficulty coping with changes in their lives. This model uses a problem-solving method to assist and support people in achieving an adaptive state. Roy's (1984) approach appeared to be particularly appropriate for an adolescent with a medical diagnosis of asthma who was having difficulty in adapting to various aspects of this chronic illness, especially since the nursing goal is to promote adaptation or a positive coping response to the stress encountered by the client. Roy (1984) observed the great resilience shown by children when responding to major physiological and psychological change. However she identified that this adaptation, or positive coping, was enhanced by nursing intervention that sought to support and promote this positive change.

Another reason for choosing Roy's model was the desire to discover whether the model would identify a nursing role for the school nurse in the provision of care in schools for children with asthma. According to Nash *et al.* (1985) and Sawley (1983), many problems associated with attending school have been identified by such children and their parents. Sawley argues that some children who suffer from asthma induced by exercise may be excluded from school games sessions, thus isolating them from their peers. Such isolation may lead to 'lack of confidence, depression and even long-term psychological problems'.

The subject of this care plan, a 17-year-old girl called Lucy, was experiencing such problems. She feared that she would be excluded from a school ski trip because of others' anxieties about the management of her asthma away from home in a foreign country. The use of Roy's (1984) model showed during assessment that Lucy had other anxieties, indirectly related to asthma. As was mentioned earlier, some authors argue for a link between emotional disturbance and asthmatic attacks although it must be stressed that Clark (1984) argues that 'no amount of emotional disturbance will induce asthma in a non-asthmatic person'.

It is likely therefore that a complex interplay of physical, psychological and social factors are at work in any individual with a medical diagnosis of asthma. Thus it is postulated that a model of nursing must be selected that is sensitive to this complexity.

Lucy's initial problem appeared to be that she feared that others were concerned about her physical capacity to manage the possible hazards of a school ski trip. Roy (1984) argues that although the adaptation model can be seen primarily as a systems model, it also contains interactionist levels of analysis because the nurse uses her own and others' interaction with the patient to manipulate elements of the system or the environment. Roy (1980) also sees the individual as a biopsychosocial being because of the presence of biological, psychological and social components or systems which determine behaviour. Therefore, in the first instance, it appeared possible that by being aware of these interactionist elements within the systems model, the nurse might find an approach to meet Lucy's needs more comprehensively than by merely concentrating on physiological factors.

Description of Roy's Adaptation model

Having explained why this particular model was chosen for this care plan, the main elements of the Roy Adaptation model will be examined.

The basic outlines of the adaptation model were first published by Roy in 1970 and the model has been expanded and refined over the years. Roy (1970) argues that any concept of nursing should begin with the patient who is the recipient of nursing care. She views the individual as both a biopsychosocial being and an adaptive system (1984). According to Roy (1971) the individual is in 'constant interaction with the changing environment' and uses both innate and acquired mechanisms which are biological, psychological and social in origin to adapt to stimuli or stressors encountered. These mechanisms are termed the regulator and the cognator subsystems.

The regulator subsystem involves biological processes, such as neurological, chemical and endocrine activities which allow the individual to cope with changes in the environment. The cognator subsystem involves psychological processes which allow the individual to deal cognitively and emotionally with stimuli encountered. However Roy (1984) indicates that there is still much work to be undertaken on the theory of the cognator and regulator processes.

According to Roy (1980) the activity of adaptation is seen in the behavioural responses demonstrated in four areas, called modes of adaptation. These are identified as the physiological, self-concept, role function and interdependence modes. Tedrow (1984) compares the four modes of adaptation with Maslow's (1954) hierarchy of needs, which ascend from basic biological needs to more complex psychological motives that become important only after the basic needs have been satisfied. Tedrow argues that Maslow's notion of self-actualisation equates with the notion of mastery in all four modes in the Roy Adaptation model.

The adaptation concept used by Roy originated in the work of Helson (1964), a physiological psychologist, who argued that individuals' ability to adapt is dependent upon the stimulus to which they are exposed and their adaptation level when coping with change. According to Helson the adaptation level at any given instant is a weighted geometric mean of all stimuli, past and present, and their effects on the attribute being judged. Similarly Roy (1980) argues that the adaptation level is made up of the pooled effect of three classes of stimuli: focal, contextual and residual. Focal stimuli are those immediately confronting the individual, and residual stimuli are beliefs and values developed from past learning (contextual stimuli are all the other stimuli present). According to Roy and Roberts (1981) adaptation is the process of responding positively to the influences of these three sets of stimuli and each individual has a variable level of coping ability. Responses which fall within this zone are positive but those which fall outside the adaptation zone will be negative and maladaptive. Roy (1984) argues that each individual copes differently with changes in health status. Only by clearly identifying each individual's level of adaptation and coping abilities can the nurse intervene to promote adaptation.

An example of the use of Roy's model is that of Burns and Kinney (1983) in a study of a patient with asthma. Burns (1983) points to the shortcomings of using the medical model approach to care for a patient with chronic asthma who smokes. For example a medical model might value effort being spent on discovering the ideal bronchodilator drug whilst undervaluing attempts to identify the reasons why the person continues to smoke.

Burns and Kinney (1983), while managing the patient's urgent physiological needs as a matter of priority, used Roy's model to assist and support the patient in improving coping skills by the use of such methods as counselling and patient teaching.

Roy (1984) considers that to evaluate an individual's current level of adaptation it is necessary for the nurse to assess behaviour in each of the adaptive modes. This then is the first level assessment. However, in an example of the use of Roy's model in the care of a man following a myocardial infarction, Webb (1985) argues that it may be impossible to neatly separate the modes because each influences the other and are thus part of the patient as a whole. In Roy's (1984) view, behaviour is assessed by means of the nurse's skill

in observation, ability to measure internal and external responses and skill in interviewing. Roy (1984) argues that generally the nurse ascertains jointly with the patient whether the behaviour is adaptive or ineffective although detailed information about how this is achieved is lacking.

Although the nurse is interested in maladaptive behaviours because of the wish to change them to adaptive behaviours, Roy (1984) emphasises that the nurse should also pay attention to adaptive behaviours because these should be maintained especially if threatened by changing influencing factors. A similar view is that of Martens (1986) who argues that it is important to identify strengths as well as problems in order to value an individual's contribution to adaptation.

Having decided which behavioural responses are causing concern, Roy (1984) suggests that the focal, contextual and residual stimuli contributing to each behavioural response are identified in a second level assessment. Based on this assessment, the nurse makes a nursing diagnosis which according to Roy (1980) might be one of the problems of adaptation or a 'statement of relationship between the behaviour and the impinging stimuli'. In Roy's (1984) view nursing diagnoses, once formulated, should be placed in a hierarchy of importance. Bower's (1977) criteria for determining the importance of patients' problems are suggested by Roy (1984) for use in deciding this hierarchy of diagnoses. These criteria are: firstly, problems 'which threaten the survival of the individual, family, group or community'; secondly, problems which 'affect the growth of the individual, family, group or community'; thirdly, problems which affect the 'continuation of the human race or of society'; and lastly, those problems which affect the 'attainment of full potential for the individual or group'.

According to Roy (1984) the goal of nursing intervention is usually to maintain and enhance adaptive behaviours and change maladaptive behaviours to adaptive ones. Therefore goals should be statements of behavioural outcomes of nursing care for the patient. Moreover, whenever possible, these goals should be agreed by the patient and nurse together.

In Roy's view nursing intervention centres on

managing the focal, contextual and residual stimuli. However since the focal stimulus is thought to be the primary cause of the behaviour it should be manipulated first. If this is not possible then the appropriate contextual or residual stimuli may be manipulated.

Finally, Roy (1984) argues that effectiveness of nursing intervention is evaluated. Formative evaluation refers to whether or not the goals set during the planning of nursing care have been achieved or, in terms of the adaptation model, whether the patient is exhibiting adaptive behaviour after nursing intervention has occurred. Roy (1984) suggests that to decide if a goal has been achieved, the nurse uses the same skills to gather data as in the first and second level assessments. Based on this evaluation, modifications may be made to the care plan or new priorities may be set.

Evaluating the use of Roy's model in planning the care of a girl with asthma

Lucy's nursing care will now be analysed and evaluated within the context of the nursing process and the Roy Adaptation model of nursing.

Using the framework of Roy's model, behaviour was first systematically assessed in each of the adaptive modes (Fig. 2.1). It was found that some influencing stimuli were identified simultaneously with behaviours in the first level assessment, especially in the self-concept mode, but in the interests of clarity these stimuli have been documented separately in the second level assessment (Fig. 2.2).

Assessment took place with Lucy in the medical room at school. Further data was obtained from her mother and staff at the school. Crow (1979) argues that additional sources of information should be utilised when assessing a patient's needs.

For the sake of brevity, and to avoid repetition, where a problem has been identified in the first level assessment, the second level assessment is immediately discussed although it was not actually carried out until some days later.

Although initially Lucy appeared to have prob-

lems in the physiological mode because of asthma, when the self-concept mode was assessed these apparently physical problems also affected Lucy's self-concept. According to Buck (1984) the nurse draws on an understanding of growth and development, learning theory and theories of self-concept and social interaction when assessing behaviour in the self-concept mode. According to Roy (1980) the self-concept mode has two major components, the physical self and the personal self. Rambo (1984) argues that the physical self is concerned with how an individual feels about his or her body, its various parts, control over its function and his or her mental image of it. Although an attempt was made to use Buck's (1984) notion of subdividing the physical self into body sensation and body image, and subdividing the personal self into self-consistency, self-ideal and moral-ethical-spiritual self, physical self and personal self appeared to be so intertwined as to be inextricable. Therefore, these components were considered together although the component self-ideal appeared to have separate characteristics.

The apparently physiological problems of short stature and small breast development were identified as focal stimuli in the self-concept mode where a problem of low self-esteem was noted. Driever (1984) argues that self-esteem is closely related to all aspects of the self-concept. According to Cooley (1902), Mead (1934) and Sullivan (1953), the formation of a concept of self is primarily influenced by the individual's perception of how they are viewed by others. In addition, according to Goffman (1963) a disability such as chronic asthma may stigmatise an individual in the eyes of others.

It was Lucy's perception that others treated her as a child. This might have been a response to her short stature and lack of physical development but it clearly affected Lucy's perception of self.

The work of Nuwayhid (1984) is useful when considering the role function mode. According to Nuwayhid the term 'role' is the title given to an individual as well as the behaviours that society expects an individual to perform to maintain the title. Nuwayhid argues that role performance is an individual's observed behaviours deemed appropriate by society to maintain his or her title.

Fig. 2.1 First level assessment, 5th March

PHYSIOLOGICAL MODE	
Exercise and rest	Enjoys and participates in games and sports. Enjoys swimming and cross country running. Appears to push herself to participate at times. Wants to go on school ski trip. Sleep sometimes disturbed by wheezing.
Nutrition	No apparent problem.
Elimination	No apparent problem.
Fluid and electrolytes	No apparent problem.
Breathing	Medical diagnosis of asthma since age of 2 years. Occasional wheezing.
Sensory regulation	Vision: wears spectacles. Hearing: no apparent problem. Speech: no apparent problem.
Endocrine regulation	Age 17 years – periods started. Small breast development.
Growth	Height: 1.47 metres, small stature. Weight: 32.66 kilograms. Abnormal growth velocity medically discounted.
SELF-CONCEPT MODE	
Physical and personal self	Low esteem – Lucy does not like her appearance. Feels 'too small'. Disappointed she has not grown more. Disappointed she still has asthma. Dislikes being treated as a child. Sometimes feels uncomfortable with others because of wheezing. Feels she is a strong person because of being made to cope by her mother.
Self-ideal	Short-term: Wants to go on school ski trip to Italy – anxious that she will not be allowed to go. Long-term: Wants to be a teacher. Would like asthma to cease.
ROLE FUNCTION MODE	Feels some anxiety about approaching adulthood. Concerned that people often treat her as a child. Says she has never been allowed to think of herself as sick – her mother has always encouraged her to cope. Wants to join in all school activities but thinks staff feel she should be less physically active.
INTERDEPENDENCE MODE	Gets on well with peers at school but sometimes refuses invitations for out of school activities because of possible wheezing. Likes to keep up with peers in games and sport. Some friction between Lucy and her mother – Lucy feels she is old enough to make her own decisions.

Furthermore, an individual needs to know who he or she is in relation to others in order to act appropriately.

Lucy's primary role may be determined by her age, sex and developmental stage. Therefore Lucy's primary role was that of a 17-year-old girl approaching adulthood. Erikson (1968) argues that the ability and opportunity to adopt certain roles help an individual develop a sense of identity. For Lucy, the behaviour of others towards her was producing role conflict. On the one hand she was approaching adult life but on the other, those around her perceived her as a child. Therefore, a problem within the role function mode was that certain roles were difficult for Lucy to adopt.

Tedrow (1984) argues that the interdependence mode is that in which the needs for affection are met and individuals experience a sense of feeling adequate through satisfying relationships with others. Lucy's 'affectional adequacy' (Tedrow, 1984) was assessed by the observation of behaviour in two areas described by Tedrow of a person being either a recipient or a contributor of love, respect and value.

Once behaviours have been identified in each mode, second level assessment takes place (Fig. 2.2). This, in Rambo's (1984) view, is completed when the nurse has identified the stimuli which

Fig. 2.2   Second level assessment, 19th March

Mode	Focal stimuli	Contextual stimuli	Residual stimuli
PHYSIOLOGICAL			
Exercise and rest			
Pushes herself to take part in sports (Lucy does not see this as a problem).	Wants to be like her peers.	All her peers take part in sports.	Believes she should push herself. Her mother has always encouraged her to cope.
Sleep sometimes disturbed (Lucy does not see this as a problem).	Wheezing	Asthma	Believes everyone with asthma wheezes.
Breathing			
Occasional wheezing (Lucy does not see this as a problem).	Asthma	Takes medication to control wheezing.	
SELF-CONCEPT			
Low self-esteem. Dislikes her appearance (seen as important by Lucy).	Small stature Small breasts	Other girls of her age are taller and have larger breasts.	Believes she is unattractive because she is short. Believes it is important for girls to develop 'normal' breasts.
Dislikes being treated like a child.	Thinks of herself as adult.	Age 17 years. Feels she is a strong person.	Believes people treat her as a child because she is short.
Embarrassed when she wheezes in company of others.	Feels different	Wheezing	
Disappointed she has not grown more.	Small stature	Puberty	Lucy thought that at puberty she would grow taller.
Disappointed she still has asthma.	Continuing asthma	Puberty	Lucy's mother had asthma which improved markedly at puberty.
Anxious that she may not go on school trip (Lucy's major problem at present).	Wants to be like her peers. Does not want to feel restricted.	Lucy feels able to cope with trip. Is confident her medication controls wheezing adequately. Feels able to make her own decisions.	Believes her parents and her teachers won't let her go.

Fig. 2.2 (continued)

Mode	Focal stimuli	Contextual stimuli	Residual stimuli
ROLE FUNCTION			
Anxious about approaching adulthood.	Rarely treated as an adult.	Often treated as a child.	Believes that at 17 years she should be treated as an adult.
Role conflict	Staff think she should not be as physically active as peers.	Other girls participate in all games and sports.	Lucy wants to join in all activities.
Lucy has rarely adopted the sick role (Lucy does not see this as a major problem).	Mother has always encouraged her to cope positively with asthma.	Mother had asthma as a child.	Lucy feels she has sometimes been made to go to school even when feeling unwell.
INTERDEPENDENCE			
Lucy finds it harder to get on with her peers out of school.	Lucy is sometimes rather aggressive when unsure of herself or troubled by wheezing.	Lucy gets embarrassed when she wheezes. Generally enjoys being with friends.	Believes that asserting herself will make up for her small stature.
Friction between Lucy and her mother.	Lucy feels she is an adult.	Lucy's mother does not always treat her like an adult.	

relate to the adaptation problems during the first part of the assessment process.

Lucy's problems in the self-concept and role-function modes seemed to centre on her perception of self. According to Norris and Kunes-Connell (1985) there may be a relationship between level of self-esteem and such factors as 'physical and mental health problems and functional role capacity'. This would appear to confirm the identification of both physical attributes and role conflict as stimuli affecting Lucy's poor perception of self.

According to Meisenhelder (1985) the nurse may enhance an individual's self-esteem by conveying both verbally and non-verbally that he or she is positively valued by the nurse. The effectiveness of this positive reinforcement can be increased by extending the number of times the nurse is in contact with the patient. Furthermore, Cohen and Lazarus (1979) argue that sharing information may aid the patient's understanding of his or her situation, thus alleviating anxiety and assisting a move towards positive adaptation. Therefore to enhance Lucy's self-esteem the nurse met her at regular intervals to allow Lucy to talk about her anxieties. The nurse's role was to show interest and to be willing to answer questions.

Since Lucy's self-concept was influenced by her perception of how others viewed her, and particularly by restrictions placed upon her, it seemed necessary for the nurse to discuss with Lucy's mother and teacher the feasibility of Lucy joining the ski trip. It also seemed appropriate to discuss asthma with Lucy's teachers to help them understand her present difficulties. According to McGovern (1981) and Colver (1984), teachers may be anxious about allowing children to participate in activities such as sports. McGovern (1981) argues that teachers who are fearful may convey fear to their pupils. Thus educating teachers about positive ways of encouraging children with asthma to participate in school activities such as sport may minimise such anxiety in teachers and consequently in their pupils.

Roy (1984) sees evaluation of the effectiveness of nursing intervention as the final step of the nursing process. To determine the effects of nursing intervention, the school nurse identified Lucy's behaviour in the four modes as the time for the

Fig. 2.3   Care plan, 19th March

Nursing diagnosis	Goals	Date	Intervention	Evaluation	Modification
Low self-esteem.	Lucy to adapt to her small stature and small breast development by stating some positive things about her appearance.	16.4	School nurse will provide opportunities for Lucy to express her feelings about herself and her appearance and will encourage Lucy to identify positive things about herself. (Meisenhelder, 1985; Cohen and Lazarus, 1979)	Lucy continues to feel trapped in a vicious circle in which her small stature means she is treated like a child and she hates to be small.	School nurse and Lucy to explore other ways of improving Lucy's body image. To consider a new hair-style. More time needed for Lucy to talk to school nurse.
	Lucy to become more self-aware and to alter her own behaviour to avoid being treated like a child.	14.5	Lucy and school nurse to talk about behaviours that lead to Lucy being treated as a child, and to discuss non-aggressive ways of being assertive.	Lucy acknowledges verbally that aggressive behaviour in the past has been childlike at times.	
Anxiety caused by uncertainty about school trip.	Lucy will be able to go on school trip.	9.4	School nurse to discuss feasibility of trip with staff and Lucy's parents.	Agreement for Lucy to go on trip if school nurse goes as well.	Staff to be better informed about asthma as discussions identified numerous misunderstand-ings about the nature of Lucy's 'condition'.
Anxious about approaching adulthood.	Lucy will adapt to approaching role of adult by expressing confidence in her own abilities.		No additional interventions at present. To be considered in 3 months.		
Role conflict about level of physical activity.	Lucy and staff will agree level of activity.	16.4	School nurse to talk to staff (especially physical education staff) about importance of physical activity for children with asthma.	Some staff expressing a greater understanding of need for physical activity.	Continue discussions. Re-evaluate 14.5.
Difficult relationship with peers especially out of school.	Lucy will adapt to her uncertainty about peer relationships as demonstrated by her accepting more invitations.	14.5	School nurse will encourage Lucy to talk about the benefits of peer support in and out of school.	Lucy has accepted more invitations from friends.	

attainment of each goal was reached, while keeping in mind Luker's (1979) view that the patient's progress should be assessed and evaluated continuously as the care plan is being evaluated (Fig. 2.3).

Initially it was felt important for teachers to develop a more realistic view of asthma and of the range of activities that Lucy might cope with and enjoy. Agreement that Lucy could join the ski trip was a major objective. This was achieved, although a compromise was reached in that Lucy was to go on the ski trip only if the school nurse went too.

The behaviour expected of Lucy as a result of nursing intervention was that she would grow in self-awareness and confidence and be capable of having relationships with both boys and girls. Furthermore, it was hoped that Lucy would gain an understanding of the various means by which she could demonstrate her role as a teenager approaching adulthood. In this way her short stature and lack of physical development might diminish in importance. Lucy eventually appeared to become more involved with her peer group socially and began to accept invitations to parties. Meetings with the school nurse allowed Lucy to discuss her feelings about issues such as asthma, small stature and relationships with others. However, more time will be required to allow her to adapt positively to being a physically small individual in an adult world.

Conclusion

Using Roy's model provided a useful framework for planning Lucy's care. It clearly identified the complex nature of human beings and reinforced the view that to consider only physiological factors when planning care is inadequate. Traditionally, nursing care for people with a medical diagnosis of asthma has focused on physical interventions often associated with drug administration. Roy's model, however, by advocating assessment in four adaptive modes, three of which centre on psychological and social concerns, ensures that physiological factors do not predominate unnecessarily.

The central tenet of Roy's model is that individuals have the capacity to adapt to or cope positively with change. As has been demonstrated here, adaptation was a necessary response by a number of people. Indeed Lucy's own adaptation would have been hampered without some change in her teacher's ability to cope positively with a pupil experiencing asthma. In addition, whilst the main objective, that of Lucy being included in the ski trip, was achieved, it was only achieved because the school nurse adapted significantly, by accompanying the trip.

Perhaps then the use of Roy's model has also highlighted the possible extent of the nurse's role. Such adaptation on the part of the nurse signifies a major departure from the role of the nurse as a physical carer avoiding close involvement with patients.

Using Roy's model has identified a role for the school nurse that emphasises liaison and negotiation between individuals. It is a role that can only be successful if both these individuals and the school nurse are willing and able to adapt to change. It is clear from this study of care that positive adaptation is frequently facilitated by increasing or up-dating people's knowledge. The school nurse must work from a sound knowledge base if she is to fulfil a key facilitatory role.

References

Anderson HR, Bailey PA, Cooper JS & Palmer JC 1981 Influence of morbidity, illness label, and social, family, and health service factors on drug treatment of childhood asthma. *The Lancet*, ii, 8254: 1030–1032.

Bower FL 1977 *The Process of Planning Nursing Care.* CV Mosby, St Louis.

Buck MH 1984 Self concept: Theory and development. In *Introduction to Nursing: An Adaptation Model*, C Roy (Ed). Prentice-Hall, Englewood Cliffs, New Jersey.

Burns MD (Ed) 1983 *Pulmonary Care: A Guide for Patient Education* (Editor's note to case study 3). Appleton-Century-Crofts, Norwalk.

Burns MD & Kinney M 1983 Use of the Roy Adaptation model in the study of a patient with asthma. In *Pulmonary Care: A Guide for Patient Education*, MD Burns (Ed). Appleton-Century-Crofts, Norwalk.

Busfield G 1982 Asthma treatment in Norway: An exercise in rehabilitation. *Nursing Mirror*, **155**, 9: 52–54.

Clark TJH 1984 *Adult Asthma.* Churchill Livingstone, Edinburgh.

Cohen SI & Lask B 1983 Psychological factors. In *Asthma*, TJH Clark & S Godfrey (Eds). Chapman & Hall, London.

Cohen F & Lazarus RS 1979 Coping with the stresses of illness. In *Health and Psychology: A Handbook*, CG Stone, F Cohen & NE Adler (Eds). Jossey-Bass, Washington.

Colver AF 1984 Community campaign against asthma. *Archives of Disease in Childhood*, **59**, 5: 449–452.

Cooley CH 1902 *Human Nature and Social Order*. Scribner's, New York.

Court Report 1976 *Fit for the Future* (Report of the Committee on Child Health Services). HMSO, London.

Crow J 1979 Assessment. In *The Nursing Process*, C Kratz (Ed). Bailliere Tindall, London.

Driever MJ 1984 Self esteem. In *Introduction to Nursing: An Adaptation Model*, C Roy (Ed). Prentice-Hall, Englewood Cliffs, New Jersey.

Erikson EH 1968 *Identity: Youth and Crisis*. Faber & Faber, London.

Goffman E 1963 *Stigma: Notes of the Management of a Spoiled Identity*. Penguin, Harmondsworth.

Gregg I 1983 Epidemiological Aspects. In *Asthma*, TJH Clark & S Godfrey (Eds). Chapman & Hall, London.

Helson H 1964 *Adaptation Level Theory: An Experimental and Systematic Approach to Behaviour*. Harper & Row, New York.

Lee DA, Winslow NR, Speight ANP & Hey EN 1983 Prevalence and spectrum of asthma in childhood. *British Medical Journal*, **286**, 6373: 1256–1258.

Levy M & Bell L 1984 General Practice audit of asthma in childhood. *British Medical Journal*, **289**, 6452: 1115, 1116.

Lewis GM & Lewis RA 1984 The place of nebulisers in childhood asthma. *Maternal and Child Health*, **9**, 1: 34–41.

Luker K 1979 Evaluating nursing care. In *The Nursing Process*, C Kratz (Ed). Bailliere Tindall, London.

Martens K 1986 Let's diagnose strengths, not just problems. *American Journal of Nursing*, **80**, 2: 192–193.

Maslow AH 1954 *Motivation and Personality*. Harper & Row, New York.

McGovern JP 1981 Chronic respiratory diseases of school-age children. In *School Nursing: Framework for Practice*, SJ Wold (Ed). CV Mosby, St Louis.

Mead D 1982 Learning to live with asthma. *Nursing Mirror*, **155**, 9: 51, 52.

Mead GH 1934 *Mind, Self and Society*. University of Chicago Press, Chicago.

Meisenhelder JB 1985 Self esteem: A closer look at clinical interventions. *International Journal of Nursing Studies*, **22**, 2: 127–135.

Nash W, Thruston M & Baly ME 1985 *Health at School: Caring for the Whole Child*. Heinemann, London.

Newby M & Nicoll A 1985 Selection of children for school medicals by a pastoral care system in an inner city school junior high. *Public Health* (The Journal of the Society of Community Medicine, London), **99**, 6: 331–337.

Norris J & Kunes-Connell M 1985 Self esteem disturbance. *Nursing Clinics of North America*, **20**, 4: 745–761.

Nuwayhid KA 1984 Role function: Theory and development. In *Introduction to Nursing: An Adaptation Model*, C Roy (Ed). Prentice-Hall, Englewood Cliffs, New Jersey.

Price B 1985 Asthma in the family. *Nursing Times*, **81**, 29: 24–26.

Price J 1984 Asthma in children: Diagnosis. *British Medical Journal*, **288**, 6431: 1666–1668.

Rambo BJ 1984 *Adaptation Nursing: Assessment and Intervention*. WB Saunders, Philadelphia.

Roy C 1970 Adaptation: A conceptual framework for nursing. *Nursing Outlook*, **18**, 3: 42–45.

Roy C 1971 Adaptation: A basis for nursing practice. *Nursing Outlook*, **19**, 4: 254–257.

Roy C 1980 The Roy Adaptation Model. In *Conceptual Models for Nursing Practice*, JP Riehl & C Roy (Eds). Appleton-Century-Crofts, Norwalk.

Roy C 1984 *Introduction to Nursing: An Adaptation Model*. Prentice-Hall, Englewood Cliffs, New Jersey.

Roy C & Roberts SL 1981 *Theory Construction in Nursing*. Prentice-Hall, Englewood Cliffs, New Jersey.

Sawley L 1983 Children with Asthma. *Nursing Mirror*, **157**, 17: 27–29.

Scadding JC 1983 Definition and clinical categories of asthma. In *Asthma*, TJH Clark & S Godfrey (Eds). Chapman & Hall, London.

Speight ANP, Lee DA & Hey EN 1983 Underdiagnosis and undertreatment of asthma in childhood. *British Medical Journal*, **286**, 6373: 1253–1256.

Sullivan HS 1953 *The Interpersonal Theory of Psychiatry*. Norton, New York.

Tedrow MP 1984 Interdependence: Theory and development. In *Introduction to Nursing: An Adaptation Model*, C Roy (Ed). Prentice-Hall, Englewood Cliffs, New Jersey.

Webb C 1985 *Sexuality, Nursing and Health*. Wiley, Chichester.

3

Care plan for a man with adult respiratory distress syndrome, using Orem's Self-care model

Sarah Gunningham

Introduction

This chapter considers the care that Paul W received when he developed adult respiratory distress syndrome (Cleeton, 1983) following admission to the intensive care unit. Paul was initially admitted to the unit for observation following resection of a primary carcinoma of the liver but developed severe bleeding and required surgical intervention on a number of occasions to control this. Following each operative procedure Paul returned to the intensive care unit. By the third admission to the unit both Paul and his wife were extremely anxious and required as much information about and involvement in planning care as possible. The care plan therefore considers the period following this third admission when Paul was intubated and ventilated.

Problems associated with mechanical ventilation

Mechanical ventilation is the most frequently used treatment in the medical management of adult respiratory distress syndrome (Cleeton, 1983). The physiological problems associated with mechanical ventilation are well documented in many texts and articles on intensive care nursing (e.g., Chalikian and Weaver, 1984; Neutze *et al.*, 1982; Tobin and Boorman, 1977). However, psychological difficulties associated with mechanical ventilation are less

frequently considered and will therefore be considered in more detail in this chapter.

Mechanical ventilation requires an airway that passes through the pharynx, larynx, and down the trachea to end just above the point at which the trachea divides into the right and left main bronchi. This tube is of great significance for most patients. By preventing airflow through the larynx and therefore also against the vocal cords, the endotracheal tube prevents the person from speaking. Tschudin (1985) has identified the difficulties experienced by many ill people being cared for in strange surroundings in making themselves understood. Such a situation is made markedly worse when, for whatever reason, patients cannot speak.

Added to this, the irritation that the endotracheal tube causes within the respiratory tract discourages people from moving more than is necessary. This loss of movement limits the use of posture, gesture, body contact and touch that are important aspects of normal non-verbal communication (Tschudin, 1985).

Loss of movement is also a contributory factor to perceptual deprivation (a reduction in the meaningfulness of stimulation) and Ashworth (1981) has emphasised how vulnerable patients in intensive care units are to such deprivation. Loss of movement decreases people's range of visual stimulation by preventing them from changing their field of vision at will. Lying supine or on either side gives a view of the ceiling or floor, and possibly the adjacent bed or wall. Sitting up increases the available field of vision, and most patients should be able to sit up for at least part of each day, provided both they and the ventilator tubing are well supported.

The endotracheal tube also makes swallowing difficult, causing the patient to require frequent oropharyngeal suction. This is an unpleasant procedure that stimulates the person to gag and cough, and this in turn may increase salivation. The difficulty experienced in swallowing, particularly in the initial period following intubation, prevents the person from eating and drinking adequately and causes loss of the sensation of taste. The reduction of airflow across the tongue may also disrupt the normal taste sensation. An inability to maintain a normal intake of fluid or diet may necessitate an intravenous infusion to maintain fluid balance and to allow for the administration of adequate nutrients. Such measures further increase immobility and dependence on nursing and medical staff.

Perceptual disturbance may also result from the nature of auditory stimulation. It would be unwise to consider hearing in the intensive care unit without also giving consideration to the high noise levels found there (Kleck, 1984). Frequently this noise level is attributed to technical machinery, but the results of several studies have found that the most disturbing auditory stimuli within intensive care units originate from communications between the staff rather than machine noise (Bentley *et al.*, 1977; Noble, 1979). Even so, the noise of intermittent airflow and ventilator alarms disturbs people's hearing and alters other, more normal sounds, thus effecting a change in people's perception of the environment. This is confirmed by Ball and Barrie-Shevlin (1985);

> the general 'hubbub' peculiar to high dependency units may override appropriate sounds normally heard by the individual.

Such perceptual disturbance, coupled with serious physical disability and perhaps involving mechanical ventilation, places considerable stress on individuals being nursed in intensive care units. This may therefore go some way towards explaining the apparent disorientation and confusion shown by many patients.

To attempt to combat some of this disturbance, nurses working in intensive care units can give priority to explaining to patients the nature of the environment in which they find themselves. Aiello (1978) has claimed that people can begin to derive meaning even from novel stimuli if adequate explanations are given. Thus the need for mechanical intervention and the nature of procedures to be carried out should all be explained clearly.

Other nursing measures may include, for example, reducing the level of artificial light. The need for careful and constant observation of people reliant on mechanical ventilation has often led to an environment permanently illumined artificially to high levels of brightness. This creates two main problems for the patient. It not only causes sensory monotony (Mackinnon-Kesler, 1983), but also interrupts normal sleep patterns and therefore increases the possibility of sleep deprivation (Fabijan and Gosselin, 1982).

Choice of Orem's Self-care model

An awareness that Paul W was vulnerable in a number of ways led to the choice of a nursing model that could address his complex needs. In addition a model was sought that would facilitate the return to independence which was hoped for and that would acknowledge the importance of sharing information with Paul and his wife in an effort to help them make sense of a strange environment.

Orem's (1980) Self-care model emphasises the existence of biological, psychological and social systems within people and is committed to the holistic nature of people (Aggleton and Chalmers, 1985). Biologically Paul had an hepatic disorder and respiratory problems, psychologically he was being cared for in a potentially frightening environment, which Thomssen (1981) has likened to culture shock, and he was socially somewhat isolated from family and friends as they lived some miles away.

Orem's model, with its aim of encouraging self-care, seemed appropriate for Paul and his wife who both wished to understand and be involved in his care. Paul's own involvement was initially limited by his physical condition but it was anticipated that he would eventually be able to achieve self-care.

Orem (1980) believes that nursing has as its special concerns

the individual's needs for self-care action and the provision and management of it on a continuous basis in order to sustain life and health, recover from disease or injury, and cope with their effects.

Orem also argues that in our society people are expected not only to be self-reliant and responsible for themselves but also for their dependants.

The notion of self-care is not unique to Orem. Blattner (1981) refers to the self-care movement and discusses the notion that few individuals have the opportunity to engage in self-care whilst in hospital even if they wish to.

Caley *et al.* (1980) suggest that the theory of self-care might eventually lead to a situation in which everyone is competent to manage their own care. This would then obviate the need for nursing. Blattner (1981) suggests that many health care professionals may feel threatened by the changes that might occur in the professional–client relationship were the client to change from passive recipient of care to active participant in care. Orem (1980) does however appear to believe that there will always be a requirement for nursing by those who are incapable of self-care, such as the unborn, the newborn, infants, children, the severely disabled, and the infirm.

The central notion of self-care within Orem's model is an important concept and highlights the fact that choosing between models of nursing should not be undertaken lightly. To choose to work with a model that advocates self-care is to accept the value of self-care. For adults in our society to be encouraged to be responsible for their own health and that of their dependants could be seen as politically attractive.

However, responsibility for health is perilously close to responsibility for ill health and care needs to be taken when using a self-care model that feelings of guilt are not engendered in those people needing nursing and/or medical attention.

Similarly a self-care model could offer a

rationale for reducing services to those considered dependent if the expectation was that adult relatives should provide care.

On the other hand Orem's model could be seen to value the contribution to care made by individuals and thus encourage health care professionals to share knowledge with patients and relatives in a more open way than is usual. Such a sharing of knowledge could pave the way for more joint decision-making about health care strategies.

Elements of Orem's Self-care model

Orem (1980) defines three types of self-care requisites, or types of self-care that individuals require, and these are shown in Table 3.1.

The universal self-care requisites show similarities to Roper's Activities of Living (Roper *et al.*,

Table 3.1   Self-care requisites (Orem, 1980)

Universal self-care requisites
These are common human needs associated with life processes and the maintenance of all human structures and their functions. There are eight universal self-care requisities.
1   The maintenance of a sufficient intake of air.
2   The maintenance of a sufficient intake of water.
3   The maintenance of a sufficient intake of food.
4   The provision of care associated with the eliminative processes and excretion.
5   The maintenance of a balance between activity and rest.
6   The maintenance of a balance between solitude and social interaction.
7   The prevention of hazards to human life, human functioning, and human well-being.
8   The promotion of human functioning and development within social groups in accord with human potential, known human limitations and the human desire to be normal. Orem calls this 'normalcy'.

Developmental self-care requisites
These are associated with human development throughout the life cycle.

Health-deviation self-care requisites
These are associated with congenital defects and the effects of disease and trauma on individual structure and functioning.

1980) and Henderson's (1966) Fundamental
Needs. The inclusion of developmental self-care
requisites supports the view that Orem's model can
be considered alongside other developmental
models.

Orem (1980) suggests five ways in which nurses
may act to implement care: by doing or acting for
another; by guiding or directing another; by
providing physical and/or psychological support;
by providing an environment which encourages
development; and by teaching.

She also defines three broad categories of
nursing intervention. These range from wholly
compensatory care offered to people unable to
engage in any form of deliberate action, through
partly compensatory care for people who are able to
make observations, judgements and decisions about
self-care but cannot perform the necessary actions,
to supportive-educative care for people who can
perform the required actions but need guidance
and supervision to make decisions about how and
when to act.

Patient profile

Paul W was a 37-year-old married man with two
daughters aged 9 and 16 years. His admission to
the hospital where this care plan was used resulted
from a referral and he was many miles from home.
His wife stayed locally throughout his time in
hospital, his daughters being cared for near their
home by relatives.

Four months prior to the commencement of this
care plan Paul had developed very itchy skin which
in spite of medication was severely disrupting his
sleep. Two weeks later Paul had yellowing of the
whites of his eyes and his skin had a deep yellow
coloration. His urine was dark yellow and his stools
were light in colour and difficult to flush away.

About a month after this a hilar cholangiocarci-
noma was removed with partial hepatectomy and
hepatojejunostomy. During the following three
weeks five further operative procedures were
undertaken:

(i)   laparotomy and splenectomy;
(ii) laparotomy and ligation of bleeding points;
(iii) vagotomy and pyloroplasty;
(iv) right hepatic lobectomy;
(v)   cholangiojejeunostomy.

During the vagotomy and pyloroplasty Paul had a
cardiac arrest which was thought to have been
caused by either stimulation of the vagus nerve or
by hypovolaemia. At the time of the cholangiojejeunostomy Paul developed laboured breathing and
was thought to have adult respiratory distress
syndrome necessitating intubation and ventilation.
It is at this point that Paul was readmitted to the
intensive care unit and the care plan described in
this paper commenced.

Discussion

The assessment of Paul's needs and the planning of
his care were organised around Orem's eight
universal self-care requisites (Fig. 3.1). Paul's
ability to be self-caring was severely impaired due
to his physical problems but it was not found
necessary to gather information about specific
health deviation self-care requisites, or to do more
than recognise Paul as an adult who appeared to
have developed in a similar way biologically, socially
and psychologically to many other adults. Thus a
detailed assessment of Paul's developmental self-
care requisites was not carried out. Such an
emphasis on the universal self-care requisites was
probably reasonable given the short stay that was
anticipated in the intensive care unit.

The care plan that follows (Fig. 3.2) does not
include all the care that Paul received. Many of the
interventions associated with Paul's physical needs
have been omitted, for example care associated
with hygiene needs and mouth care. These are not
considered unimportant but are not as necessary
for the discussion as other aspects of the care given.

The choice of a self-care model for a patient in
an intensive care unit may seem unusual. However,
frequently patients in such units are there as a
result of an acute episode of a physical nature and
as such may be unable to be self-caring for a very
limited period.

The use of a self-care model for Paul was
advantageous in a number of ways. Firstly, it helped

Fig. 3.1 Investigative procedure: Paul W, aged 37

Self-care requisites	Current self-care state	Reason for self-care deficit	Potential for re-establishing self-care/ additional data
Universal			
1 Maintenance of a sufficient intake of air.	Paul is unable to maintain a sufficient intake of air unaided. Mechanical ventilation in progress. Apical chest drain already in position. Unable to cough.	Adult respiratory distress syndrome causing breathing difficulties. Semi-conscious state inhibiting coughing. Pneumothorax reducing lung capacity. Semi-conscious. Sedated.	Should re-establish self-care. Has required mechanical ventilation before for a short period but re-established self-care with little difficulty.
2 Maintenance of sufficient intake of water.	Paul is unable to maintain a sufficient oral intake of water. Intravenous infusion in progress via left subclavian vein.	Imposed restriction on oral intake. Semi-conscious state. Recent abdominal surgery.	Should re-establish self-care. Favourite drink is weak tea. History of alcohol abuse in the past. (From medical notes).
	Mouth very dry.	Unable to take oral fluids.	In the past has found ice lollies help to moisten his mouth.
3 Maintenance of sufficient intake of food.	Paul is unable to maintain a sufficient oral intake of food. Intravenous infusion in progress to provide 4000 calories per 24 hours.	Imposed restriction on oral intake. Semi-conscious state. Recent abdominal surgery.	Difficult to assess the potential for eventually eating and absorbing adequate nutrients. Estimated weight 70 kg. Has lost 10 kg over last 3 months.
4 Provision of care associated with eliminative processes and excretion.	Paul is unable to provide all care needed. Urinary output insufficient (less than 30 ml per hour). Intravenous dopamine in progress. Urinary catheter *in situ* (Foley, size 14).	Low blood pressure. Poor renal perfusion.	Should re-establish self-care.
	Bowels not open for three days.	Paralytic ileus.	
	Naso-gastric tube in position.	Paralytic ileus.	

Fig. 3.1   (continued)

Self-care requisites	Current self-care state	Reason for self-care deficit	Potential for re-establishing self-care/additional data
5 Maintenance of a balance between activity and rest.	Paul unable to control level of activity and amount of rest. Sedated with an Omnopon infusion.	Semi-conscious. Difficult to assess Paul's awareness of his surroundings.	Prior to recent admission Paul led an active social life to which he should be able to return. Spends most evenings at the local pub where he drinks at least 4 pints of beer and occasionally ½ bottle of whisky.
6 Maintenance of a balance between solitude and social interaction.	Paul is unable to interact socially with staff or visitors. It is not possible for Paul to be left alone. His wife talks to him frequently.	Semi-conscious. Unable to communicate verbally. Paul is dependent on mechanical ventilation so cannot be left alone.	Paul's wife spends much of her time at his bedside. Paul liked her to be there prior to recent surgical intervention and seemed reassured by her presence.
7 Prevention of hazards to human life, human functioning and human well-being.	Paul is at risk from both physical and psychological hazards, as detailed above.	Unable to breathe unaided; unable to take adequate nutrients orally; unable to control what is happening to him.	Should re-establish self-care ability to function physically. Difficult to predict psychological outcome at this stage. Paul is a Roman Catholic.
8 Promotion of normalcy.	Paul is not able to function at a physical level that will sustain life. Therefore at present not able to meet psychological or social needs (Maslow, 1970).	Adult respiratory distress syndrome. Physiological and safety needs cannot be met unaided.	Paul's life-style is one that he should be able to resume. He is a self-employed picture framer and works as an accountant as well.

to focus care on the abilities that Paul had before his current health problems. This served as a constant reminder of the desired outcome of care – that Paul should return to as near a normal life-style as possible. This was important for both the staff and for Paul's wife. Particularly when a person is unconscious, it is easy for nurses to forget the person involved and his or her capabilities and aspirations. In this way care can become routinised and lose sight of the individual.

However, for relatives and friends it is the unconscious person who is unusual and the person they knew may seem almost forgotten. His wife was helped by the emphasis on long-term goals which specified desired outcomes that saw Paul returned to a self-caring adult whom she could recognise and identify with.

In addition the wholly compensatory system of nursing as described by Orem (1980) is very appropriate for an intensive care setting. Added to this is the notion within the model that nursing care must be available for those who cannot meet their self-care requirements safely. This is frequently a feature of patients requiring wholly compensatory care and Paul's need for mechanical ventilation was not because he could not breathe at all but because

Fig. 3.2 Care plan (LT = long term)

Problem/need	Goal	Intervention	Evaluation
Paul is unable to breathe unaided.	Paul will be able to breathe normally (LT).		
Paul needs all care associated with mechanical ventilation.	Paul will be safe from the complications of mechanical ventilation and will maintain an airway.	Endotracheal tube in position to maintain airway. Tube to be tied and supported to prevent movement and accidental disconnection. Cuff of tube to remain inflated to prevent air leaks and inhalation of secretions (Shafer *et al.*, 1979; Janowski, 1984). Tube to be kept patent by suction and 2-hourly instillation of saline (Oh, 1985). Nurse to remain with Paul at all times to observe for adequate ventilation.	Paul's airway has been maintained. Remains ventilated. For possible extubation tomorrow.
Paul is unable to cough.	Paul will regain ability to cough (LT).		
	Paul will not retain sputum and secretions.	Tracheal aspiration to be carried out 2-hourly (preceded by 'bagging' 4-hourly) and as necessary. Paul to be turned from side to side to prevent stasis of secretions.	Paul's chest sounds clear. Some sputum is blood-stained.
	Paul will not develop a chest infection as demonstrated by absence of pathological micro-organisms in his sputum.	Tracheal aspiration to be carried out using aseptic technique (Grossbach-Landis and McLane, 1979). Sterile gloves to be worn (Wilson, 1985). Ventilator tubing and humidifier to be changed every 48 hours (Wilson, 1985). Sputum specimens to laboratory on Mondays, Wednesdays and when extubated.	Sputum specimen sent. Results awaited. Sputum does not look infected.

Fig. 3.2   (continued)

Problem/need	Goal	Intervention	Evaluation
Paul needs care associated with apical chest pain.	Paul will have full expansion of right lung within 36 hours, demonstrated by chest X-ray.	Chest drain to be observed for signs of patency and for 'bubbling'.	Chest X-ray shows some reduction in size of pneumothorax. Continue to observe chest drain.
	Paul will not experience pain or undue discomfort from drain.	Omnopon infusion to be maintained as per medical regime. Paul to be observed for signs of restlessness.	Difficult to assess presence or absence of pain. Paul is not restless but is heavily sedated.
Paul is unable to take fluid or food orally.	Paul will resume self-care ability to take adequate nutrition orally (LT).		
	Paul will be adequately hydrated as demonstrated by urine output of over 30 ml per hour.	Intravenous infusion to be maintained as per regime. (2500 ml per 24 hours).	Urine output remains low (less than 30 ml per hour). Intravenous dopamine continues.
	Paul will receive 4000 calories per 24 hours.		Calorific input achieved. Medical staff considering the need for insulin supplements because of high glucose input.
Paul is unable to move at will.	Paul will regain ability to maintain balance between activity and rest (LT). Paul will not develop skin redness.	Paul's position to be changed 2-hourly (to include sitting up). Passive movements to be performed to Paul's limbs.	Difficult to assess ability to move due to sedation. Some skin redness apparent on left hip.
Paul is unable to communicate verbally. In the past he has needed to retain some control by hearing explanations of what is happening.	Paul will be able to verbally communicate. Paul will have all care explained to him.	Nurses to explain care to Paul and to his wife. Paul's wife to talk to Paul about what is happening. Nurses to consult with Paul's wife about his needs as she may interpret non-verbal communication more accurately.	Explanations are being given. Impossible to evaluate what Paul hears or understands.
Paul is physically and psychologically at risk.	Paul will be able to prevent hazards himself (LT). Paul's safety to be maintained by others (primarily nurses).	Nurses to carry out care as detailed above and to remain with Paul at all times. Roman Catholic priest to be contacted and asked to visit.	Little sign of improvement in Paul's consciousness level. Remains ventilated.

he could not maintain safe levels of blood gases.

Intensive care units are also care settings that are particularly unusual in terms of the environment. The effect that this might have on patients' sensory input has already been mentioned. It is helpful therefore to work with a model of nursing that emphasises the notion of being normal (or normalcy).

One of the ways in which Paul's need to feel normal was addressed was by the sharing of information with him and his wife. This also enhanced their ability to look towards self-caring as an ultimate goal. During the periods of care that preceded this care plan, both Paul and his wife had sought information about the care being offered to him. By this means they had been able to take part in decision-making about the various operative procedures. To take part in decision-making is a crucial aspect of self-care.

The importance of sharing information, even with a patient whose ability to respond in a way that is meaningful to the nurse is limited, cannot be overstated. Clifford (1985) has drawn on the work of Seligman to highlight an important aspect of caring for those who are mechanically ventilated. She argues that the feelings of helplessness which may assail the sedated person who is mechanically ventilated may be overcome by careful explanation about the return to normal breathing that is anticipated. Her work would seem to reinforce the view that a self-care model might be useful in intensive care settings if it helps to focus on desired outcomes of self-care and encourages nurses to share these with both patients and relatives.

The contribution of Orem's self-care model to the care of Paul W has been discussed. Perhaps it is most valuable in an intensive care setting because its emphasis on an ultimate goal of a return to self-care helps nurses, patients and relatives to acknowledge the transitory nature of much intensive care.

References

Aggleton P & Chalmers H 1985 Orem's self-care model. *Nursing Times*, 81: 36–39.

Aiello J 1978 The concept of sensory deprivation. *The Australian Nurses' Journal*, 7, 10: 38–40.

Ashworth P 1981 Nursing care in the ICU. *Nursing Times*, 77: 1063–1064.

Ball C & Barrie-Shevlin P 1985 Sensory deprivation. In *High Dependency Nursing*, D O'Brien & S Alexander (Eds). Churchill Livingstone, Edinburgh.

Bentley S, Murphy F & Dudley H 1977 Perceived noise in surgical wards in an intensive care area: An objective analysis. *British Medical Journal*, 2, 6101: 1503–1506.

Blattner B 1981 *Holistic Nursing*. Prentice-Hall, Englewood Cliffs, New Jersey.

Caley JM, Dirksen M, Engalla M & Hennrich ML 1980 The Orem self-care nursing model. In *Conceptual Models for Nursing Practice*, JP Riehl & C Roy (Eds). Appleton-Century-Crofts, Norwalk.

Chalikian J & Weaver TE 1984 Mechanical ventilation – Where it's at, where it's going. *American Journal of Nursing*, 84, 11: 1372–1379.

Cleeton C 1983 Shock lung. *Nursing Times*, 79: 27–29.

Clifford C 1985 Helplessness: A concept applied to nursing practice. *Intensive Care Nursing*, 1: 19–24.

Fabijan L & Gosselin MD 1982 How to recognise sleep deprivation in your ICU patient and what to do about it. *Canadian Nurse*, 78, 4: 20–23.

Grossbach-Landis I & McLane A 1979 Tracheal suctioning: A tool for evaluation and learning needs assessment. *Nursing Research*, 28, 4: 237–242.

Henderson V 1966 *The nature of nursing: A definition and its implications for practice, research and education*. Macmillan, New York.

Janowski MJ 1984 Accidental disconnections from breathing systems. *American Journal of Nursing*, 84, 2: 241–244.

Kleck HC 1984 ICU syndrome: Onset, manifestations, treatment, stressors, and prevention. *Critical Care Quarterly*, 6, 4: 21–28.

MacKinnon-Kesler S 1983 Maximising your ICU patient's sensory and perceptual environment. *Canadian Nurse*, 79, 5: 41–45.

Maslow AH 1970 *Motivation and Personality*. Harper & Row, London.

Neutze JM, Moller CT, Harris EA, Horsburgh MP & Wilson MD 1982 *Intensive Care of the Heart and Lungs*. Blackwell Scientific Publications, Oxford.

Noble MA 1979 Communication in the ICU: Therapeutic or disturbing? *Nursing Outlook*, 27, 3: 195–198.

Oh TE 1985 *Intensive Care Manual*. Butterworths, Sydney.

Orem DE 1980 *Nursing: Concepts of Practice*. McGraw-Hill, New York.

Roper N, Logan W & Tierney AJ 1980 *The Elements of Nursing*. Churchill Livingstone, Edinburgh.

Shafer KN, Sawyer JR, McLusky AM, Beck EL & Phipps WJ 1979 *Medical-Surgical Nursing*. CV Mosby, St Louis.

Thomssen R 1981 Psychological aspects of intensive care units, or, culture shock in hospitals. *The New Zealand Nursing Journal*, 74, 9: 26–27, 34.

Tobin G & Boorman J 1977 Nursing care of a ventilated patient. In *Tracheostomy and Artificial Ventilation in the Treatment of Respiratory Failure*, SA Feldman & BE Crawley (Eds). Edward Arnold, London.

Tschudin V 1985 Communication. In *High-Dependency Nursing*, D O'Brien & S Alexander (Eds). Churchill Livingstone, Edinburgh.

Wilson AP 1985 Pseudomonas infection and the ventilated patient. *Intensive Care Nursing*, 1: 2, 107–110.

4

Care plan for a man following a spontaneous haemopneumothorax, using Johnson's Behavioural Systems model

Valerie Newton

Introduction

The nursing care that is planned for patients who have sustained pneumothoraces or haemopneumothoraces has, according to Allan (1985), changed greatly over the last few years. Allan argues that much of this change has been dependent on factors ranging from physicians' wishes to hospital policy.

It is against such a background that this chapter considers the nursing care offered to one man following spontaneous haemopneumothorax. Some relevant literature is reviewed concerning nursing care and the use of Johnson's behavioural model is described.

The patient, Peter Jones, was a 19-year-old man, employed as a postman. He sustained a spontaneous haemopneumothorax following a fall from his motorbike and was admitted to the intensive care unit where he remained for 48 hours.

Review of literature

A review of current literature concerning the nursing care of patients with pneumothoraces or haemopneumothoraces reveals several factors. Firstly, much of the literature (Meador, 1978; Lane, 1979; Bricker, 1980; Cohen, 1980; Erickson, 1981; Franco, 1983; Mims, 1985) is North American. Secondly, in much of the care described there appears to be no model of nursing on which the nursing care is based. Taken together these two

factors point to a paucity of literature from this country evaluating care for patients with pneumothoraces or haemopneumothoraces using a model of nursing.

Much of the literature (e.g., Meador, 1978; Cohen, 1980; Erickson, 1981; Horsington, 1984; Allan, 1985; Mims, 1985) regarding care of a patient with a pneumothorax follows a similar theme. There is a brief resumé of the anatomy and physiology of the lungs and surrounding organs, a definition of pneumothorax, a list of types of pneumothoraces and their causes, the signs and symptoms likely in a person with a pneumothorax and some technical information regarding underwater seal drains and the principles governing their use. Other literature, for example that of Welch and Lennox (1979) and Tang (1983), is very medically oriented, because the authors are physicians and are not therefore writing specifically about nursing care.

Some salient points, however, may be extracted from the literature cited above. For example, Allan (1985) stresses the value of giving information to patients with a pneumothorax and explaining carefully any procedures planned. Such recommendations are supported within other nursing contexts (e.g., Ashworth, 1978; Wilson-Barnett, 1979; Gardiner, 1980).

Allan (1985) also advocates regular assessment of the patient although he appears not to link this to the nursing process. As Yura and Walsh (1983) suggest, assessment alone is of little value but as part of the nursing process it is crucial.

Some literature has sought to address the controversy surrounding the clamping of underwater seal drains (e.g., Nichol, 1983) and such studies are useful in raising nurses' awareness of the issues involved. However, a plan of nursing care should focus on the individual rather than on one technical aspect of care. Horsington (1984) recognises this and goes further in that patient behaviour such as sleep and activities to prevent boredom are considered.

A move away from nursing care organised largely on the basis of medical signs and symptoms demands a model of nursing. Johnson's model seemed attractive because it focuses on behaviour (which usually informs a nursing assessment) and yet recognises the fundamental human capacity for homeostasis. Henderson's (1960) model might appear suitable in that it highlights biological changes but it was felt that it might prove insensitive to aspects of the patient's behaviour motivated by psychological and social factors.

Johnson's Behavioural Systems model of nursing

According to Fawcett (1984) the rudimentary idea of Johnson's conceptual model was evident in a 1959 article. However, the more complete model was presented in 1980 in Riehl and Roy's established text on models of nursing (Riehl and Roy, 1980). It is therefore a model which has undergone a period of development although published examples of its use in practice remain relatively recent. (e.g., Damus, 1980; Grubbs, 1980; Haladay, 1980; Small, 1980 – all in Riehl and Roy, 1980).

It is also Johnson's definition of a model of nursing that has served to highlight certain characteristics of models. For example Johnson argues that models should be based on understandings which are 'scientifically based' and that the ideas within models should be used to inform nursing practice. She also acknowledges that to choose a particular nursing model involves nurses working with a particular set of values. While on the face of it such concerns are commendable, Johnson offers

little evidence in support of the development of her model. However, the notion of behaviourism has a long tradition within psychology and methods of changing people's behaviour are not new within health care. Furthermore, nursing assessment relies heavily upon observation and such assessment therefore *observes* behaviour.

Johnson's model is a systems model which supports the view that the whole person is something more than the sum of his or her parts (or, in Johnson's model, subsystems). Some of the literature mentioned above appears to view a part of the person, namely the presence of an underwater seal drain, as more important than the whole. It was hoped, by selecting a model with an emphasis on behaviour rather than on physiological functioning alone, that a more individualised and sensitive plan of care could be offered.

Johnson (1980) advocates that nursing makes a contribution to health care by facilitating effective behavioural functioning in the patient before, during and following illness. In order to achieve this facilitation the model focuses on the individual who is regarded as a behavioural system. According to Johnson, all patterned, repetitive and purposeful ways of behaving that characterise a human's life are considered to make up his or her behavioural system.

To explore the key elements of Johnson's model, a format based on that suggested by Aggleton and Chalmers (1984) will be used. Thus the model will be examined in terms of what it has to say about the nature of people, the environment, nursing and the reasons why nursing intervention is required. In addition, the nature of assessment, planning, intervention and evaluation will be considered.

According to Loveland-Cherry and Wilkerson (1983), people in Johnson's model display actions and behaviours which are controlled and regulated by biological, psychological and social factors. Although Canner and Watt (1986) argue that the idea of regarding 'man' as a behavioural system is unique to Johnson, they acknowledge the contribution of work on adaptation, behaviour modification, social learning, sensory stimulation and motivation.

Johnson suggests that people may be regarded therefore, as behavioural systems made up of a number of subsystems which perform specialised functions necessary for survival. These subsystems are the attachment (sometimes known as the affiliative) subsystem, the dependency subsystem, the ingestive subsystem, the eliminative subsystem, the sexual subsystem, the aggressive subsystem and the achievement subsystem. Details of the way in which the subsystems may motivate individuals towards certain behaviours are tabulated in Table 4.1.

It is noticeable that Johnson has included the sexual subsystem, an aspect of human functioning to which explicit reference is frequently omitted (e.g., Henderson, 1960; Roper *et al.*, 1980). Other authors have however been critical of some of Johnson's ideas. Fawcett (1984) for example questions the heavy biological focus within Johnson's description of the ingestive and eliminative subsystems.

The whole human system, and thus all the subsystems, require what Johnson has called sustenal imperatives. These are environmental factors necessary for adequate functioning and comprise protection, nurturance and stimulation. It is likely therefore that nursing intervention planned within the context of Johnson's model will involve nurses in altering the amount of protection, nurturance and stimulation available to patients.

So far mention has been made of the functioning of the subsystems. Johnson (1980) however, conceptualises each subsystem as having four structu-ral elements, namely drive, set, choice and action. The drive (or sometimes the goal) of any subsystem is the motivating force which encourages certain behaviours. Set is concerned with individuals' predispositions to act in certain ways, and develops through experience and learning. Choice identifies each individual's repertoire of behaviours from which choices are made. Johnson has argued that it is rare for people to utilise all the behavioural alternatives available to them and the notion of set is consistent with this. However, she appears to support the view that, when needed, behaviours are often to be found within a person's repertoire even though they may appear not to be preferred. Finally the action of each subsystem is the observable behaviour.

Johnson argues that the subsystems tend to be self-maintaining and that as long as conditions in both internal and external environments are orderly, interrelationships tend to be harmonious. However, if these conditions are not met, as may occur during periods of illness, then malfunction may occur. This is demonstrated by erratic, disorganised and dysfunctional behaviour. However, Fawcett (1984) is critical that Johnson does not define illness or wellness. This must be seen as a major criticism as without a clear definition it is difficult to do more than borrow a definition from the medical model.

Nursing is necessary according to Johnson as an

Table 4.1   Johnson's seven subsystems (adapted from Grubbs, 1980)

Subsystems	Behavioural motivation
Attachment/affiliative	Towards the need for security. Also associated with the needs of social inclusion and the formation and maintenance of social links within society.
Dependency	Towards the need for nurturance, approval, attention, recognition or physical assistance.
Ingestive	Towards appetite and thirst satisfaction including amount and type of food and circumstances in which eating takes place.
Eliminative	Towards the need to eliminate.
Sexual	Towards the needs of procreation and gratification. Includes but is not limited to courting or mating.
Aggressive	Towards the need for protection and preservation of the individual and society.
Achievement	Towards the need to have control over oneself and one's environment. Involves a range of cognitive and physical skills.

external regulatory force acting to preserve the organisation and integration of behaviour at an optimal level for an individual whose behaviour constitutes a threat to physical or social health. The goal of care is to restore, maintain or attain behavioural system balance and stability of the highest possible level for the individual.

Although Johnson does not specifically advocate the nursing process as a means of implementing her model, the work of Grubbs (1980) does offer some useful guidelines.

Assessment aims to establish an accurate picture of a person's behaviour both currently and prior to the need for health care. This information can be gathered from many sources, ranging from the patient and family to other health team workers. The importance, however, of the data gained from the patient cannot be overstated.

Assessment can usefully be regarded as having two stages. The first stage involves an examination of patient behaviour with a particular emphasis on identifying instability within the subsystems. The nurse may spend some time establishing the patient's usual pattern of behaviour in order to make comparisons and may also consider any past instances when the patient required nursing intervention for some reason.

If there exists a potential or actual problem then a second level of assessment is made. During this, the nurse tries to discover the cause of any imbalance and is likely to consider the supply of sustenal imperatives and the structural elements of the subsystem(s). Information may be sought about the source and sufficiency of sustenal imperatives for each subsystem and in particular a careful search is made for factors that might be restricting the patient's behaviour. For example, illness sometimes isolates an individual from the company of others. This may cause some imbalance in the dependency subsystem.

During this second stage of the assessment process, the nurse will also gather data about the structural elements of the subsystems. A problem in one subsystem may sometimes be due to incompatibility with another subsystem. Thus, if behaviour is overwhelmingly motivated by a desire to be totally in control (goal of the achievement subsystem), this may affect the likelihood of

establishing successful social relationships (goal of the attachment subsystem).

Grubbs (1980) supports the view that problems identified will usually stem from an environmental excess or deficiency, or will arise within the structure of a subsystem.

Following problem identification, planning should take place to set goals and specify the expected behaviours that will indicate goal achievement. Using Johnson's model will tend to focus goals on the restoration of stability within and between the subsystems.

Nursing intervention needs to respond to the cause or causes of the problem and may therefore focus on the supply of sustenal imperatives or on the structural elements of the subsystem.

Four modes of intervention are described (Johnson, 1980), which reinforces the notion that nurses have choices to make about the ways in which they can intervene. According to Johnson, nurses may restrict, defend, inhibit or facilitate. For example, if an individual is experiencing an excess of protection from well-meaning friends and relatives, the nurse may seek to limit or restrict their involvement to restore stability in the patient's achievement subsystem.

If the major cause of the problem is found to be structural, the nurse may seek to expand the behavioural choices open to the patient, alter the subsystem set, change the behaviour (action) or strengthen the drive. Nurses may adopt the role of facilitator to enable individuals to learn new behaviours.

Grubbs (1980) stresses the importance of previously specified goals when trying to evaluate the success of nursing intervention. She favours the use of both long and short-term goals and appears to acknowledge that, whereas long-term goals are likely to indicate eventual subsystem equilibrium, short term goals are the means of individualising care. Formative evaluation can then be organised around the achievement of goals with particular note taken of the expected behavioural outcomes.

Fawcett (1984) is sceptical that although both Johnson (1980) and Grubbs (1980) claim the use of this conceptual model encourages nursing actions that result in personal satisfaction for the nurse and improved patient care, as yet no empirical evidence to support this is available. Evaluation of the use of Johnson's model for Peter Jones should contribute to the debate.

Evaluation of the use of the model

Johnson's (1980) behavioural model of nursing appeared to be a feasible and generally successful model on which to base Peter's care, although the limited time span over which it was used (approximately 48 hours) necessarily means that evaluation here must be somewhat tentative.

Peter was admitted with a medical diagnosis of a right haemopneumothorax and three fractured ribs on the right side. He was in need of urgent medical and nursing intervention and it would have been comparatively easy to focus nursing attention on physiological concerns. However, using Johnson's model provided the opportunity to also consider psychological and social aspects affecting Peter's care.

It had initially been planned to record observed behaviour and action in each subsystem separately. However, during assessment (Fig. 4.1) it became clear that this was introducing unnecessary repetition as the action of each subsystem *is* the observed behaviour.

Gathering data around each of the structural components of the subsystems proved more useful than had been anticipated. This assessment provided much pertinent information for later goal

Fig. 4.1   Assessment of Peter Jones, aged 19

Action	Drive	Set	Choice	Sustenal imperatives
Attachment subsystem				
Friendly and talkative with nursing staff. Appears to get on well with parents and two younger sisters. Says he has many friends.	Likes to be with family and friends.	Would usually seek out companionship.	Rarely chooses to be alone.	Gains nurturance and security from being with known others. Visiting to be encouraged if Peter wishes this.
Dependency subsystem				
Is physically unable to care for himself because of pain and presence of underwater seal drains. Asking for explanations and reassurance.	Seems to accept need for temporary physical dependence on others.	Is normally self-caring.	Does not wish to be dependent on nursing care for long. Able to accept this in the short term.	Pain and presence of underwater seal drain. Needs protection from too much activity which might exacerbate pain.
Ingestive subsystem				
Breathing is very painful due to right haemopneumothorax and 3 fractured ribs. Feels short of breath. Looks cyanosed. Respiratory rate 22 per minute.	To be able to breathe in sufficient oxygen.	Usually breathes without difficulty.	Choice restricted. Presently having to take rapid shallow breaths due to inspirational pain.	Pain.
Feels nauseated.	Needs to eat and drink adequately.	Usually eats and drinks as desired.	Would choose not to eat and drink at present.	

Fig. 4.1 (continued)

Action	Drive	Set	Choice	Sustenal imperatives
Eliminative subsystem (after 3 hours)				
Has an underwater seal drain to help lung re-expansion.	To breathe normally.	Usually breathes normally. Presence of underwater seal drain is a new experience.	Peter is unsure how much he can move about while drain *in situ*. Dislikes presence of drain.	Possibly too much stimulation from concern about presence of underwater seal drain.
Dislikes using urinal.	Needs to empty bladder.	Does not usually use a urinal.	Would choose to go to the lavatory.	
Sexual subsystem				
Not assessed. Did not appear relevant during acute time in unit.				
Aggressive subsystem				
Very agitated and distressed at times. Feels frightened by breathing difficulty and intensive care environment.	Self-protection.	Would usually be able to breathe easily. No previous experience of intensive care unit but has been in hospital before.	Accepts admission to intensive care unit but is unsure how to behave.	Intensive care environment is too stimulating. Care needed to ensure Peter feels safe (protection).
Achievement subsystem				
Unable to be physically independent. Asking for lots of information about medical treatment, nursing care and possible length of hospital stay.	Needs information to allow sense of control.	Usually in control of own physical activities and knowledgeable about what is happening to him. Finds asking questions helps him to feel some control.	Can adapt to physical dependence at least in the short term.	Having to cope with many novel experiences. Give information and answer all questions as means of nurturance.

setting and care planning. For example, identification of normal behavioural preferences or predispositions (set) often became the precursor of the planned goals. To a lesser degree this was also true of the factors identified as part of the choice of each subsystem. A careful study of the care plan illustrates the use of assessment data in this way.

It should not be assumed that gathering information about the structural elements of the subsystems was easy. What appeared to be helpful however, was to pose questions related to Peter's normal behaviour in order to understand the set of each subsystem, and to ask about what he would choose to do and how much he could cope with in his present situation in order to discover the extent of his behavioural repertoire (choice).

The notion of determining the supply and sufficiency of sustenal imperatives also proved difficult. However, some were identified with reasonable confidence and these are documented on the care plan (Fig. 4.2). What was significant, and gave a degree of confidence in the information

Fig. 4.2   Care plan for Peter Jones

Nursing diagnosis	Goal	Nursing action	Evaluation
Day 1			
Peter is feeling breathless and looks cyanosed. (Dominance of ingestive subsystem.)	Peter will feel less breathless and will look a pinker colour.	Provide the necessary mask for Peter to receive oxygen at 4 litres/min. Assist doctor during procedure to insert drain to right side of chest. Record respiratory rate, pulse rate and BP $\frac{1}{2}$-hourly. Observe underwater seal drain for signs of adequate functioning hourly.	Peter says he feels less breathless. Respiratory rate now 16 per minute. 300 ml blood and pus drained in first $1\frac{1}{2}$ hours.
Breathing is painful. Movement painful. (Over-stimulation from internal environment.)	Breathing will become less painful. Movement will become less painful.	Administer prescribed analgesia. Make Peter as comfortable as possible in bed.	Peter says he can breathe with less pain. Movement remains painful.
Peter likes to feel in control. (Drive of achievement subsystem.)	Peter will express satisfaction at extent of explanation he receives.	Answer all Peter's questions honestly. Explain all nursing care before and during nursing interventions.	Peter says he feels happier now he knows what is happening.
Agitated by present situation. (Over-stimulation from external environment especially ICU.)	Peter to be less agitated.	Reduce environmental stimulation as much as possible by keeping noise to a minimum and reducing lighting. Explain the environment to Peter if he wishes.	Peter still agitated at being in ICU. Dislikes unfamiliar surroundings and feels uneasy. Wants to go to a general ward.
Day 2			
Persisting pain on breathing and when moving.	Pain to be within acceptable limits for Peter.	Administer prescribed analgesia. Ensure maximum comfort in bed.	Pain improved and within acceptable limits.
Peter is breathing more deeply and maintaining a pink colour without additional oxygen.	Peter's breathing to remain unchanged when underwater seal drain clamped.	Clamp drain. Observe for any change in respiratory rate or breathing depth. Observe facial colour.	Peter continues to breathe deeply and remains a pink colour.
Remains unhappy to be in intensive care.	Peter to be transferred to a general ward.	Discuss Peter's concern with care team to facilitate early transfer.	Transferred to general ward.

recorded, was that these sustenal imperatives began to suggest ways and means of intervening. Indeed, some general guidelines for Peter's care emerged which were very helpful although they did not link to specific problems. Rather they showed ways in which Peter's normal life-style and supply of sustenal imperatives could be maintained. A good example of this was Peter's need for the companionship of known others which highlighted the importance of visitors to him.

It will be noted that Peter's particular breathing difficulties have been located within the ingestive and eliminative subsystems. This is not explicitly advocated by Johnson but is supported by the notion of taking in something (adequate oxygen) and getting rid of waste (products of respiration). Grubbs (1980) has documented a similar use of these subsystems.

Certain observed behaviours or actions noted during assessment did not directly call for nursing intervention while Peter was in ICU. In particular, although Peter disliked using a urinal, he was prepared to put up with the embarrassment for a limited time. Similarly no direct intervention took place to control Peter's nausea. It was felt that this would resolve once the pain and distress he was experiencing were reduced by other means. In the event no problems related to eating and drinking occurred. Johnson's model is a systems model which therefore supports the view that the elements contributing to the nature of people are interrelated. Thus it is not unusual for intervention in one subsystem to affect behaviour in another.

Finally, Johnson's emphasis on behaviour needs further consideration. It would be unjust to identify Johnson's model too readily with behaviourism and the development of techniques to change people's behaviour. Certainly behavioural outcomes are anticipated when using the model. However, whereas behaviour modification techniques seek to alter behaviour and show minimal interest in the cause of the behaviour, Johnson stresses the need to search for causative factors. Indeed the emphasis during assessment on discovering information about sustenal imperatives and about the structural elements of each subsystem clearly directs the nurse towards the importance of identifying possible causative factors.

It is hoped that this use of Johnson's model will encourage debate and evaluation about its appropriateness as a basis for planning and delivering nursing care. The model appears to have been successfully used already by Haladay (1980), who documents the assessment of health status and the choice of nursing interventions made for a variety of children requiring care. Rawls (1980) used the model to plan nursing care for an adult following leg amputation, and Skolny and Riehl (1984) also comment favourably on the use of the model in practice. Further careful research is clearly needed but, as Fawcett (1984) has argued, the model offers an approach to care which focuses on behaviour rather than a disease process and such a concept deserves attention.

References

Aggleton P & Chalmers H 1984 Models and theories – Defining the terms. *Nursing Times*, 80, 36: 24–28.

Allan D 1985 Chest tube patients. *Nursing Times*, 5, 81: 24–25.

Ashworth P 1978 Communication in the ICU. *Nursing Mirror*, 146, 7: 34–36.

Bricker PL 1980 Chest tubes: The crucial points you mustn't forget. *Registered Nurse*, 43, 11: 21–26.

Cohen SC 1980 Programmed instruction: How to work with chest tubes. *American Journal of Nursing*, 80, 4: 685–712.

Canner SS & Watt JK 1986 Behavioural system model. In *Nursing Theorists and Their Work*, A Marriner (Ed). CV Mosby, St Louis.

Damus K 1980 An application of the Johnson Behavioral System model for nursing practice. In *Conceptual Models for Nursing Practice*. JP Riehl & C Roy (Eds). Appleton-Century-Crofts, Norwalk.

Erickson R 1981 Chest tubes: They're really not that complicated. *Nursing (US)*, 11, 5: 34–43.

Fawcett J 1984 *Analysis and Evaluation of Conceptual Models of Nursing*. FA Davis, Philadelphia.

Franco LA 1983 Double-barrelled therapy for pulmonary crisis. *Registered Nurse*, 46, 11: 44–48.

Gardiner B 1980 Our responsibilities to the person, beside the Respirator. *New Zealand Nursing Journal*, 71, 2: 7–11.

Grubbs J 1980 The Johnson Behavioral System model. In *Conceptual Models for Nursing Practice*, JP Riehl & C Roy (Eds). Appleton-Century-Crofts, Norwalk.

Haladay B 1980 Implementing the Johnson model for nursing practice. In *Conceptual Models for Nursing Practice*. JP Riehl & C Roy (Eds). Appleton-Century-Crofts, Norwalk.

Henderson V 1960 *Basic Principles of Nursing Care*. International Council of Nursing, London.

Horsington V 1984 Pneumothorax. *Nursing Mirror*, 158, 6: 39–41.

Johnson DE 1980 The Behavioral System model for nursing. In *Conceptual Models for Nursing Practice*, JP Riehl & C Roy (Eds). Appleton-Century-Crofts, Norwalk.

Lane CS 1979 Skilled care for the pneumothorax patient. *Journal of Nursing Care*, 3, 2: 16–17.

Loveland-Cherry C & Wilkerson SA 1983 Dorothy Johnson's Behavioral System model. In *Conceptual Models of Nursing: Analysis and Application*, JJ Fitzpatrick & AL Whall (Eds). Robert J Brady Co, Maryland.

Mims BC 1985 You *can* manage chest tubes confidently. *Registered Nurse*, 48, 1: 39–44.

Meador B 1978 Pneumothorax: Providing emergency and long term care (with care during chest drainage). *Nursing (US)*, 8, 11: 43–45.

Nichol J 1983 Management of underwater chest drainage. *Nursing Times*, 79, 8: 58–59.

Rawls AC 1980 In *Analysis and Evaluation of Conceptual Models of Nursing*, J Fawcett (Ed) (1984). FA Davis, Philadelphia.

Riehl JP & Roy C 1980 *Conceptual Models for Nursing Practice*. Appleton-Century-Crofts, Norwalk.

Roper N, Logan W & Tierney A 1980 *The Elements of Nursing*. Churchill Livingstone, Edinburgh.

Skolny MS & Riehl JP 1984 In *Analysis and Evaluation of Conceptual Models of Nursing*, J Fawcett (Ed) (1984). FA Davis, Philadelphia.

Small B 1980 Nursing visually impaired children with Johnson's model as a conceptual framework. In *Conceptual Models for Nursing Practice*, JP Riehl & C Roy (Eds). Appleton-Century-Crofts, Norwalk.

Tang HL 1983 *Laboratory and diagnostic tests with nursing implications*. Prentice-Hall, London.

Welch J & Lennox SC 1979 Treatment of spontaneous pneumothorax. *Nursing Times*, 75, 8: 324–326.

Wilson-Barnett J 1979 *Stress in Hospital Patients: Psychological reactions to illness and health care*. Churchill Livingstone, Edinburgh.

Yura H & Walsh MB 1983 *The Nursing Process: Assessment, Planning, Implementation, Evaluation*. Appleton-Century-Crofts, Norwalk.

5

Care plan for a child with a ventricular septal defect, using Neuman's Open Systems model

Kate Harris

Introduction

The care offered to a family with a child awaiting corrective surgery for a ventricular septal defect is discussed in this chapter, as is the Neuman (1980) Open Systems model with some of Clark's (1980) adaptations.

The care centres on three visits made by the health visitor during the pre-operative period. Post-operative care is not included due to the surgical intervention being postponed. However, pre-operative care involved some discussion of long-term goals but these will not be met until surgical operation has taken place.

The health visitor's involvement during the pre-operative phase and the anticipated involvement during the post-operative period identified the importance of interaction with the family. As is frequently the case with health visiting, contact with the family took place in their home. The family had been known to the health visitor since the birth of John in 1983 and a certain amount of information was already available. The health visitor had therefore had the opportunity to establish a positive relationship during this time.

The development of nursing models is a recent occurrence, and may be linked to nurses becoming more aware of their status and wanting professional recognition. Many nurses believe that the development of nursing should be towards a profession seen as complementary rather than subordinate to the medical profession. In order to be recognised as professionals, nurses and health visitors require an accepted theoretical framework on which to base their practice. This, coupled with changes in health care, makes a move from disease-orientated to person-orientated systems of care attractive to nurses and health visitors.

Choice of model

Neuman's (1980) model with Clark's (1980) adaptation was chosen as the theoretical framework for planning care because, firstly, a positive relationship between health visitor and client cannot develop without an awareness of the client's perception of his or her life. Secondly, within the assessment process advocated by Neuman, stressors are identified according to the client's perception of a situation and compared with those stressors identified by the health visitor. Finally, a health visitor works mainly with the well population whether her case load is predominantly families with children under five years, the elderly, or a cross section of all age groups. Such an emphasis on wellness is consistent with the framework of Neuman's model. Research into how individuals respond to stress can also be used to support the use of a nursing model that clearly sees people exposed to, and coping with, stress (or stressors).

Menzies (1960) and Lazarus (1983), for example, found that nurses exposed to stress at work often coped by using denial. A parallel can be drawn with a family facing imminent major surgery for one of its members (a stressor) which copes by denying the likelihood of the event occurring. Such denial means that the family cannot adequately prepare for the event.

A model such as Neuman's may encourage different coping strategies by offering an assessment format that values the perceptions of both clients and nurses, thus making denial difficult.

Relevant literature

Selye (1974) describes stress as 'a non-specific response' and uses the extreme emotions of joy and sorrow to demonstrate that things both pleasant and otherwise can be described as stressors. Individuals are constantly confronted by stress. Freedom from stress according to Selye (1974) would equate with death. The variety of ways in which individuals cope with stress is likely to determine the amount of involvement they have with the caring services.

In initiating interventions with the family to help them prepare for John's imminent surgery, Seligman's (1975) work on helplessness was considered. Seligman describes helplessness as the stage reached when individuals are no longer in control of a situation. Similarly, 'powerlessness' is a term used by Miller (1983) to describe the feelings of individuals who perceive their actions as having no effect on situational outcomes.

During John's stay in hospital, his parents may experience helplessness or powerlessness as they will be confronted with unfamiliar situations and equipment and staff who have had very little time in which to build a relationship with them.

According to Sundeen et al. (1981), if carers demonstrate a caring attitude this will increase individuals' security when faced with unfamiliar situations. Verbal and non-verbal communication are used to convey caring. In John's case, information on touch and familiar soothing phrases used by his parents would need to be conveyed to hospital staff. His parents could be motivated to do this by the health visitor.

It is important to consider the research by Beverley (1936) which demonstrated that children often thought they were ill because they had misbehaved. This finding has been supported more recently by Pidgeon (1978), and adds emphasis to the importance of verbal and non-verbal communication between child and carers to ensure that the child understands as much as possible about the reasons for being in hospital.

This research is useful to the health visitor in encouraging the parents to participate in the care of their child whilst he is hospitalised.

Research by Nuckolls et al. (1972) and Holmes and Rahe (1967) attempted to investigate the beneficial effects of social support when individuals are faced with stressful situations. Generally speaking, they found that the presence of social support has a beneficial effect in enabling an individual to cope more positively with stressors. This can be related to Neuman's (1980) assessment/intervention tool which requires the client and family to discuss their expectations of help from care-givers, family and friends.

Neuman's (1980) systems model of stress and reaction, with system stability as the system goal, was considered the most appropriate model to use in view of these research findings and the author's own work experience. Furthermore Neuman suggests assessment of stressors from both the client's and the health visitor's point of view and advocates a summary of impressions to help identify the differences between the two.

As health visitors practise mainly with the well population it is a vital part of their work to assess both client and health visitor perceptions of the same situation in order to plan interventions acceptable to the client or family.

Neuman's model

Gestalt theory is one of the key concepts of Neuman's model, highlighting the importance of people's perception of themselves and their surroundings and indicating that the invasion of the system by one stressor can colour people's perception of other stressors and affect their lines of resistance. Neuman's portrayal of the client system as a central core surrounded by lines of defence and resistance which can be penetrated by stressors is considered to contain basic survival features unique to that client (Fig. 5.1).

Neuman views the person as being made up of four distinct variables which interrelate. These are the physiological, psychological, sociocultural and developmental variables. Reaction to stressors is influenced by intra-, inter-, and extrapersonal factors, with the resistance of the client system depending on the interrelationship of the four variables.

The interaction between people and their environments is important within Neuman's model and Clark's (1980) adaptation, given that human beings live in a world where they are constantly subjected to stimuli of various kinds. Consequently, perception develops as a way of organising and interpreting these stimuli into potential or actual stressors.

In visits made to this family, Neuman's assessment/intervention tool based on the health care systems model was used and Clark's (1980) representation of health visitor–client consultation was incorporated.

Clark's representation contains key words which, once used on a regular basis, may provide a useful format for future contact between health visitor and client. These key words could incorporate Neuman's suggested assessment/intervention tool once the health visitor is familiar with the theoretical basis of care (Fig. 5.2).

Application of Neuman's model to practice is not widely documented. Craddock and Stanhope (1980) have reported an incomplete study by Home Healthcare Agency in the United States which used Neuman's assessment/intervention tool. Initial results indicate concern about the reliability of the questions as they are worded in assessment. In an earlier study, Pinkerton (1974) expressed similar concerns.

In using Neuman's model as a basis for care, the wording of these questions has been adapted to reflect the client's use of language and level of understanding. Clark's (1980) representation of health visitor–client consultation, based on her tape-recordings of home visits, proved useful in

making these adaptations.

Neuman's model can be compared with the nursing process and the principles of health visiting as identified by the Council for the Education and Training of Health Visitors (1977), in that the main elements of each are present, yet the evaluation stage is poor. This may be due to the tendency of health visitors to dwell on collection and assessment of data, which, following negotiation with the client may result in no action.

Clark (1980) criticised traditional health visiting as 'being all assessment without implementation' as health visitors spent most of their time collecting data to compare with the 'norm' in order to detect deviation. Therefore Clark decided not to systematically collect this information, and she only recorded a small part of the available background data. She also found in her own health district that very few health visitors kept a 'family' card for every family visited.

Furthermore Clark (1983) observed that health visitors are under pressure to use 'outcome evaluation' which is used in medical evaluation. A problem arises for those health carers concerned with prevention in that the outcome looked for is often that something does not happen. This results in a rather different emphasis from much medical and nursing evaluation.

A vital part of the health visitor's work concerns the ability to form relationships. Clark (1980) demonstrates this in her health visitor–client consultation by incorporating the negotiation of a relationship within the initial contact, together with the health visitor stating the purpose of her visit (Fig. 5.2). Initiation of contact can be by either the health visitor or the client.

Research has emphasised the importance the consumer places on a 'friendly approach' by the health visitor in her initial contact with the family. Field *et al.* (1982), in a small-scale survey of mothers, found that health visitors were received positively by the consumer when their approach was friendly. Orr (1980) asked consumers to list 'the ideal attributes of a health visitor', and this resulted in 'friendly' being considered the most important attribute. A survey by Clark (1984) supported Orr's findings.

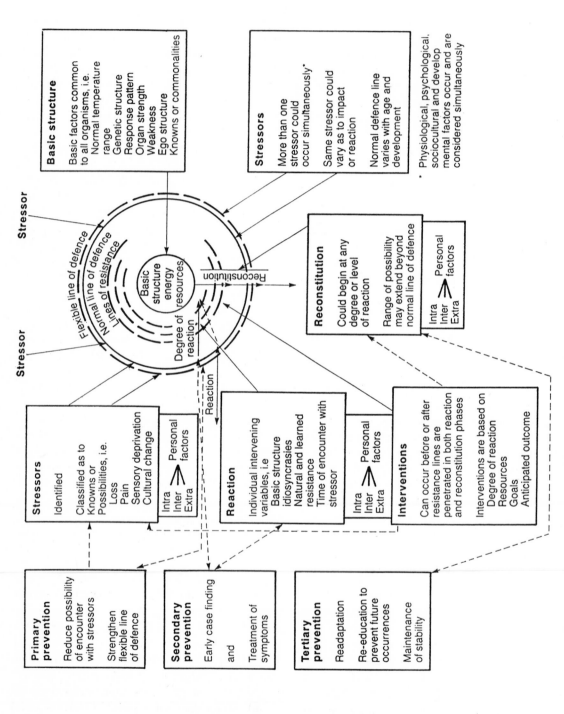

Fig. 5.1 Diagrammatic representation of Neuman's systems model. Adapted from Neuman and Young (1972)

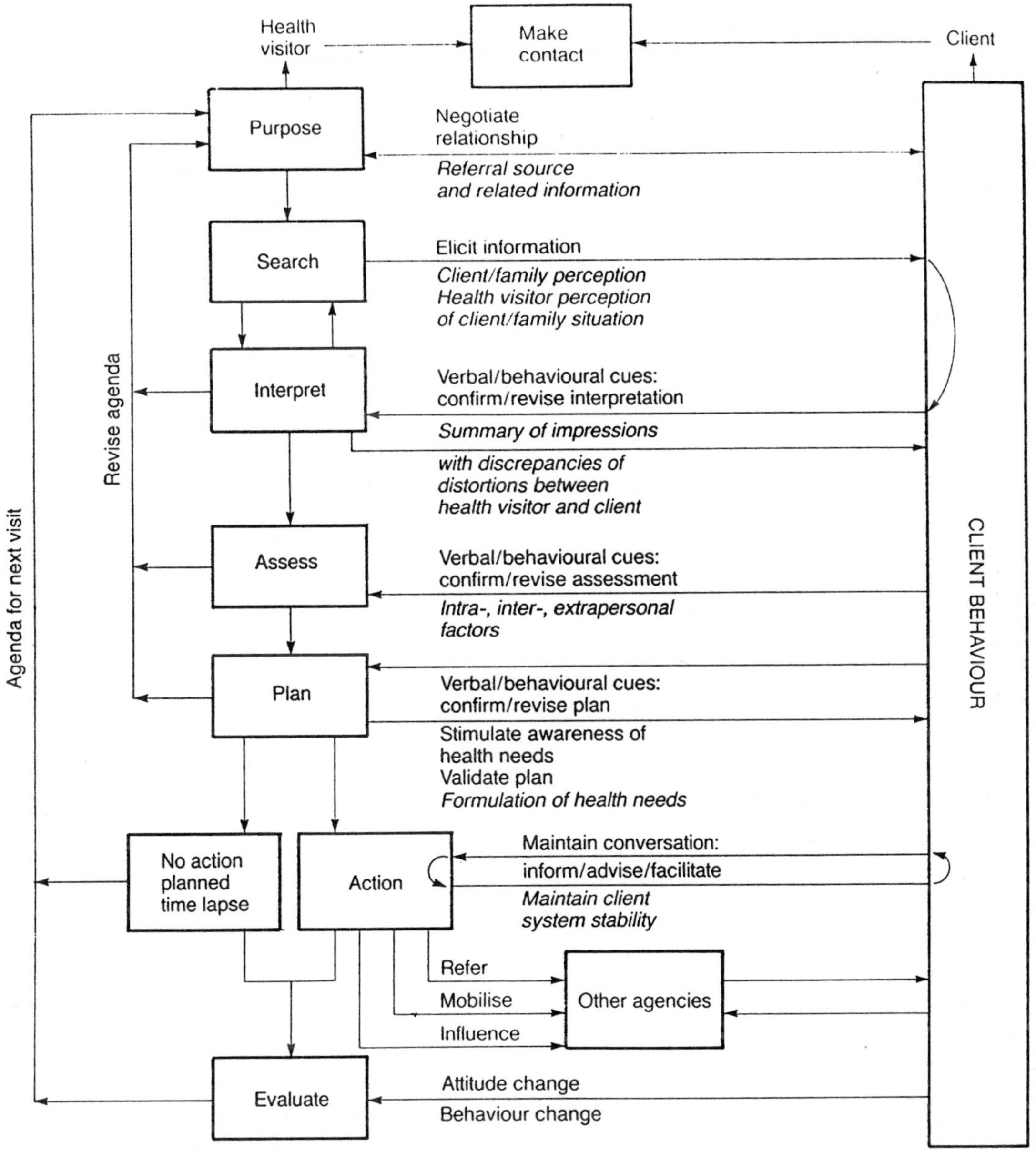

Fig. 5.2 Health visitor–client consultation, combining Clark's (1980) model of health visitor activity with Neuman's (1980) assessment/intervention tool (the latter given in italics). Adapted from Clarke (1980) with permission from *Health Visitor*

Use of Neuman's model

A relationship had already been formed between the family in this study and the health visitor due to her contact with them following John's birth.

The family structure consisted of Mr X, Mrs X, Tony (Mrs X's son by her first marriage) and John, Mr X's only child.

Contact with the family was initiated by the health visitor for two reasons: firstly, to check John's developmental progress and secondly, to initiate discussion about John's heart surgery which was expected to take place before his third birthday.

At the age of two years John's development had been assessed at the Well Baby Clinic by the community physician. He noted that John's speech had not developed very well since his assessment at 18 months old. Following this earlier assessment he had been referred to the speech therapist for advice.

Although John's development was the focus of the home visit by the health visitor, it was made explicit that there was a twofold purpose in the visit. Both parents were present during the visit.

Assessment

John's indistinct speech, lack of interest in toilet training, and possessive attitude to his mother were classified as potential family stressors. The impending heart surgery was considered an actual stressor affecting the family's view of John in general.

John's erratic appetite was also a potential stressor, as his parents wanted him to be strong enough to cope with the expected surgery and believed his food intake was important in achieving this. This illustrates how the actual stressor of the diagnosed ventricular septal defect has coloured the parents' view of their child. The potential stressor of John's occasional tantrums also illustrates this, as the parents were concerned at the possibility of him being uncooperative with hospital staff.

In order to plan future care, assessment of intra-, inter- and extrapersonal factors identified as stressors was also undertaken with Mr and Mrs X, using the family care plan.

According to Neuman (1980) intrapersonal factors are those arising from within the individual, interpersonal factors being outside individuals.

Neuman (1980) classifies intrapersonal factors as physical, psychosociocultural and developmental, with Clark (1980) emphasising the use of verbal and behavioural cues to confirm or revise assessment. These factors are categorised with health needs in the care plan.

John's physical intrapersonal factor of a medically diagnosed ventricular septal defect was assessed as instigating a special need in the care plan.

Developmentally it was noted that John's motor and hand/eye coordination were within normal limits, requiring no action other than reassessment at the age of three.

Intrapersonal factors relating to the parents are demonstrated with the health need 'psychological', as Mrs X was concerned about John's personality changing should he have a blood transfusion.

Assessment of interpersonal factors relates to resources and relationships that could influence intrapersonal factors. Tony's paternal grandmother is seen as a source of help to the family whilst John is in hospital. Her help will make it possible for Mrs X to stay with John during his time in hospital. The speech therapist, health visitor and surgeon also are perceived by the family as resources.

Assessment of extrapersonal factors includes knowing that Mr X is a milkman, and that his wife works five nights a week at a supermarket. This necessitates them both liaising with their employers about John's expected surgery in order for them to be absent from work. Health service resources are assessed particularly in relation to the parents' concern about the risk of AIDS.

Planning and intervention

In planning care Neuman (1980) follows assessment with 'formulation of the problem', but as many of the stressors are potential rather than actual it would seem more appropriate to talk in terms of formulating health needs. These needs can be prioritised by establishing short and long-term goals, remembering that 'action' or 'no action' is carried out to maintain client-system stability.

Neuman (1980) considers intervention to be via one of three preventive modes, primary intervention being the one which most relates to health visitor activity.

The short-term goals planned with Mr and Mrs X involved immediate action by the health visitor to contact the speech therapist. It was also planned that the parents should avoid the intake of food being an issue between them and John. The concern expressed by Mr and Mrs X about the suitability of blood donors prompted the health visitors to supply information on the risk of contracting AIDS from donated blood.

Long-term goals included agreement on delaying toilet training, on John having outings with his father, and on the parents avoiding provocative situations where possible. In the long term, the health visiting goal was to strengthen resistance factors by supplying correct information, and supporting the family before, during and after John's proposed surgery.

Desensitising noxious stressors, such as Mrs X's fear of a change in John's personality following a blood transfusion and the fear of AIDS, could be brought about by supplying specific information in

Fig. 5.3 Care plan: child

Name: John		Date of birth: 14.11.83		Stressors: A = actual, P = potential	
Date	Health needs	Assessment	Goal	Intervention	Evaluation
21.3	Motor development	Within normal limits.	To maintain this.	Health visitor to review when 3 years old.	
21.3	Hand/eye development	Within normal limits.	To maintain this.	Health visitor to review when 3 years old.	
21.3	Hearing/ speech development	1 Speech indistinct **P** 2 Hearing satisfactory for speech development	John to achieve satisfactory speech.	Health visitor to contact speech therapist as appointment not yet received.	Speech therapy due to start in 2 weeks. 16.6 Speech clearer.
21.3	Personal/social development	1 Not toilet trained **P** 2 Possessive attitude to mother **P** 3 Tantrums **P**	John to be toilet trained. John to become less possessive. Tantrums to become infrequent.	Parents delay toilet training until John shows interest. HV review in three weeks. Parents encourage visits by friends and relatives. Father to take John out with him.	16.6 John responds to visiting friends and relatives. Only occasionally asks for Mummy when alone with his father. Tantrums less frequent.
21.3	Nutrition	Erratic appetite **P**	John to eat only at meal times.	Parents to avoid making food an issue.	21.4 Seen at children's surgery. Now eating with rest of family without any difficulties.
21.3	Special needs	1 Diagnosed VSD **A** 2 Corrective surgery prior to third birthday **A**	Parents to prepare themselves and John for the proposed surgery. Date to be fixed for surgery.	HV will supply information on proposed surgery. HV to contact surgeon's secretary for date.	4.4 Surgeon contacted by HV. Surgeon to write to parents with necessary information. 2.5 Letter received by parents. 16.6 No date fixed for surgery. 3.9 Surgery still delayed.

Fig. 5.4   Care plan: family

Family members: Mrs X, Mr X, Tony		Dates of birth: 1960, 1957, 1978		Stresses: A = actual, P = potential	
Date	**Health needs**	**Assessment**	**Goal**	**Intervention**	**Evaluation**
21.3	Physiological	Only applicable to John. Other family members functioning normally.			
	Psychological	Mrs X anxious that John's personality will change if he has a blood transfusion **A**. Mr X uncertain about this.	Parents will be less anxious about possibility of personality change.	Health visitor to look for information on this and contact surgeon.	Surgeon contacted. 2.5 Letter received by the family. Parents feeling less anxious.
	Environmental	Family live in a 3-bedroom semi. John will be in hospital for up to three weeks following surgery. Parents have seen hospital ward where John will be and they are aware of the facilities. Mr X is a milkman **P**. Mrs X works evenings. Neither parent smokes. Family holidays planned for August.	Mr and Mrs X to have adequate leave from work when John is in hospital.	Mr and Mrs X to inform employers of John's health status. Mrs X to arrange four-week holiday whilst John is in hospital.	Both employers sympathetic to situation. Mrs X able to take four-week annual leave.
	Social relationships	Tony has regular contact with paternal grandmother. Mr X's brother and family live in the same street.	Tony to be cared for satisfactorily whilst John is in hospital.	Tony to stay with grandmother when John is in hospital.	Grandmother happy to have Tony to stay.
	Special needs	Both parents anxious about risk of AIDS if John has donated blood **A**. Parents would like to donate their own blood **P**.	Parents to be less anxious about risk of AIDS and therefore no longer wish to donate blood to John.	Health visitor to give parents information about the risk of AIDS. Health visitor to request surgeon to reinforce information about AIDS. Parents' blood to be grouped.	Parents less anxious and no longer wishing to donate blood to John. Blood grouped.
3.9	Psychological	Mrs X still anxious about blood transfusion but less so than before.	Mrs X to be less anxious.	Health visitor will continue to give support and advice over the coming months.	

an understandable form to Mr and Mrs X enabling them to be confident in their decision to proceed with surgical correction of John's ventricular septal defect.

It is interesting that a summary of impressions highlighted the discrepancy between Mrs X's knowledge of personality changes caused by blood transfusions and the health visitor not perceiving this as a potential problem. Also the parents' fear of AIDS being transmitted was very real, but the health visitor had not perceived this as a stressor.

The health visitor's perception was not the same as the parents' because she had access to up-to-date information on such issues. Consequently, together with the surgeon she was able to relate this to the parents. The parents were able to accept the information from the health visitor and surgeon, probably because they had had the opportunity to develop a trusting relationship with both health care workers over a period of time. If their son was in a life-threatening situation they both agreed that they would accept any treatment which gave some likelihood of saving his life. This highlights the tremendous responsibility health care workers have in ensuring that clients are adequately informed of possible treatments and outcomes.

John would be considered 'a high risk' according to Neuman's (1980) assessment scheme, which indicates that intervention should take place at the primary prevention level. It can be observed in the care plans (Figs 5.3 and 5.4) that intervention is not only undertaken by the health visitor, but also by the parents. This demonstrates the mainly primary preventative role of the health visitor.

Evaluation

Mrs X was seen at the children's surgery a month after the initial care plan was drawn up, and she reported John to have a good appetite and to be eating his meals with the rest of the family. This was evaluated as demonstrating that the intervention was successful and a short-term goal had been achieved. John was, however, not attending speech therapy.

As planned, the long-term goals were evaluated at a home visit three months later. The actual stressor of John's proposed surgery remained unchanged, as the family had not been given a firm date for this.

The actual stressor of a possible personality change due to transfused blood had also been relieved, together with the parents' concern about AIDS, as a result of the information from the health visitor and that contained in a letter from the surgeon to the parents. The extent of this relief would only be evident in the months following surgery, illustrating the necessity for the health visitor to maintain it as a long-term goal.

Discussion

In providing care for this family, the health visitor adopted more than one role at each contact with them. The Council for the Education and Training of Health Visitors (1977) defined the role and function of the health visitor in terms of the five main areas of prevention; early detection and surveillance of high risk groups, recognition of need, health teaching and provision of care. Four skills were also identified within the concept of the role, these being observation, developing interpersonal relationships, teaching individuals and groups, and skills of organisation and planning.

Another health visiting role suggested by the Council for the Education and Training of Health Visitors (1977) and Clark (1980) is the role of searcher, as the health visitor is searching for health needs in her work with clients. This is seen as coming before the assessment stage of the health visiting process and has been used with this family in the search for perception of stressors. This is explicit in the care plan.

The role of searcher and the use of skills in observation and listening were also important in obtaining information on social background, attitude, attempts to conceal anxiety, and the channelling of concern into an 'acceptable' area such as the child.

When first visiting the family, stating the purpose of the visit enables an initial role relationship to be negotiated between client and health visitor. How far the client participates in this negotiated relationship will affect the whole health visitor–client consultation.

The formulation of the care plan with the family might appear to be time-consuming. However, the time spent was vital in determining a pattern of care and enabling potential role conflict to be identified. The combined use of the work of Neuman (1980) and Clark (1980) enables interpretation of a summary of impressions in which discrepancies between family needs and what the health visitor considers she can offer can be explored.

By focusing on the management of John's care the health visitor was able to guide the parents into discussing their health needs in relation to those of the rest of the family. The presence of Mr X at the visit was considered beneficial by both parents as they had never actually sat down to discuss John's condition in depth. Mr X was unaware of his wife's fears. She had not shared them in order not to alarm him. Suppression of such fears, however, could have caused serious distress to all family members at a later date.

In the provision of care to this family all five functions outlined by the Council for the Education and Training of Health Visitors (1977) were used, together with those of counsellor and communicator.

Craddock and Stanhope (1980) in their recommended adaptation of Neuman's model observed that Neuman identified the health visitor as an advocate for the client and family during interaction with the health care system. 'Advocate' is defined by Kosik (1975) as a person giving support, identifying and providing for needs, and interceding in the system for the client. This is closely related to the roles defined by the Council for the Education and Training of Health Visitors (1977). With this family, the health visitor acted as advocate for them in liaison with the surgeon and speech therapist.

Clark (1984) considers it important for the health visitor to make her function explicit both to the client and herself in order to minimise dissatisfaction on the part of the client with the health care system.

In evaluating care given, it is necessary to stress the time taken in using the health visitor–client consultation which combines Neuman's assessment tool. Certain information from this family was already available to the health visitor and did not need to be collected again. Even so, it is important not to be complacent, as a family is a small social system which moves through stages in its life-cycle and will require reassessment from time to time.

In evaluating care the family were able to perceive their progress towards planned goals clearly. They found their involvement in care increased their awareness and gave them the confidence to express their feelings.

Using this model, in conjunction with the parents, helps to build up their self-esteem and feelings of worthiness as value is put on their contribution to their child's care and development. This should strengthen their resistance to other stressors which may occur as the time of John's surgery approaches.

References

Beverley BI   1936   Effect of illness upon emotional development. *Journal of Paediatrics*, 8: 534.
Clark J   1980   A framework for health visiting and the nature of health visiting activity. *Health Visitor*, 53, 11: 487–489.
Clark J   1983   Evaluating health visiting practice. *Health Visitor*, 56: 205–208.
Clark J   1984   Mothers' perceptions of health visiting. *Health Visitor*, 57: 265–268.
Council for the Education and Training of Health Visitors   1977   *An Investigation into the Principles of Health Visiting.* Council for the Education and Training of Health Visitors, London.
Craddock RB & Stanhope MK   1980   The Neuman Health-Care Systems Model: Recommended Adaptation. In *Conceptual Models for Nursing Practice*, JP Riehl & C Roy (Eds). Appleton-Century-Crofts, Norwalk.
Field S, Draper J, Kerr M & Hare M   1982   A consumer view of the health visiting service. *Health Visitor*, 55: 299–301.
Holmes T & Rahe R   1967   The social re-adjustment rating scale. *Journal of Psychosomatic Research*, 11: 213–218.
Kosik SH   1975   Patient advocacy or fighting the system. In *Contemporary Community Nursing*, B Spradley (Ed). Little Brown & Co, Boston.
Lazarus R   1983   The costs and benefits of denial. In *The Denial of Stress*, S Breznitz (Ed). International University Press, New York.
Menzies I   1960   Institutional defence against anxiety. *Human Relations*, 13: 95–121.
Miller JF   1983   *Coping with Chronic Illness: Overcoming Powerlessness.* FA Davis Co, Philadelphia.
Neuman B   1980   The Betty Neuman Health-Care Systems Model: A total person approach to patient problems. In *Conceptual Models for Nursing Practice*, JP Riehl & C Roy (Eds). Appleton-Century-Crofts, Norwalk.
Neuman BN & Young RJ   1972   A model for teaching total person approach to patient problems. *Nursing Research*, 21, 3: 264–269.

Nuckolls CB, Cassell J & Kaplan BH 1972 Psycho-social assets, life crises and the prognosis of pregnancy. *American Journal of Epidemiology*, 95: 431–441.

Orr J 1980 *Health Visiting in Focus*. Royal College of Nursing, London.

Pidgeon VA 1978 Child thought and counselling implications in hospital. *Patient Counselling and Health Education*, 1, 1: 4–7.

Pinkerton A 1974 Use of the Neuman Model in a home health care agency. In *Conceptual Models for Nursing Practice*, JP Riehl & C Roy (Eds). Appleton-Century-Crofts, Norwalk.

Roy C 1980 The Roy Adaptation Model. In *Conceptual Models for Nursing Practice*, JP Riehl & C Roy (Eds). Appleton-Century-Crofts, Norwalk.

Seligman M 1975 *Helplessness*. WH Freeman & Co, San Francisco.

Selye H 1974 *Stress Without Distress*. Hodder & Stoughton, London.

Sundeen SJ, Stuart GW, Rankin E de S & Cohen SA 1981 *Nurse–Client Interaction: Implementing the Nursing Process*, 2nd Ed. CV Mosby, St Louis.

6

Care plan for a man following a myocardial infarction, using Peplau's Developmental model

Timothy Holt

Introduction

This chapter discusses the care of Mr Thomas Fletcher, a 67-year-old man who has retired from full-time employment as a chartered surveyor but still does some work on a consultancy basis. He has been married for 45 years and lives with his wife in a large detached house which they have owned for 20 years.

Mr Fletcher and his wife have two sons who are both married with children of their own. The family appears to be very close and its members mutually caring.

Mr Fletcher is a member of several social and charitable organisations. In most cases, his membership involves his assumption of an active role such as Secretary or Treasurer. These responsibilities involve commitments of both time and energy.

His only previous experience of hospitalisation was following the diagnosis of bacterial endocarditis two years ago. He spent 9 weeks in hospital but recovered with no evident residual damage to the structure of his heart or other organs. He has no chronic medical problems and normally has no need of the primary health care team.

The day before his admission to hospital, Mr Fletcher had spent the afternoon gardening. He had needed to stop half-way through cutting a high hedge because of pain in his left shoulder and arm which he attributed to muscle strain. The pain did not completely resolve with rest and paracetamol but became much less acute. He spent the remainder of the day resting quietly and went to bed about 11 pm.

In the early hours of the next morning he was awoken by crushing central chest pain. His wife telephoned their family doctor and Mr Fletcher was admitted to hospital with a provisional diagnosis of myocardial infarction.

This example of the use of Peplau's model was somewhat complicated by the fact that Mr Fletcher was initially admitted to the hospital's coronary care unit (CCU) rather than directly to the ward on which the model was used. Mr Fletcher was in CCU for 36 hours during which time he was cared for by nurses using Henderson's Fundamental Needs model of nursing (Henderson, 1966).

When he was transferred to the ward, the possibility was considered of rationalising the care he had received in CCU in terms of Peplau's model and including it in the care plan that forms the basis of this chapter. The idea was rejected on the grounds that it would both be clumsy and might detract from the value of the care plan as a practical application of a nursing model.

It might be argued that his experience of Henderson's model and the care he received in CCU would influence Mr Fletcher's attitudes towards nursing and the care planned for him using Peplau's model. For example, he might have felt that the central concerns of assessment were sleeping habits, bowel action, micturition and mobility because of the importance allotted to these behaviours by Henderson (Riehl and Roy, 1980). To combat this potential prejudice, Mr Fletcher was given an explanation of Peplau's model that sought to acquaint him with the basic concerns and tenets of the model. He grasped the concepts of the model quickly and expressed enthusiasm about its use in the organisation of his nursing care.

This implementation of Peplau's model was undertaken on an acute medical ward. Patients of both sexes, admitted with a variety of medical diagnoses, are cared for on the ward. The nursing process forms the basis for nursing care delivered on the ward and is usually based on Henderson's model.

Review of literature

As detailed below, Peplau's model of nursing is primarily concerned with the psychoanalytical and interactionist aspects of nursing care (Meleis, 1985). For that reason, this review of literature relevant to Mr Fletcher's care will focus on psychological and sociological rather than physiological approaches to the care of patients who have suffered a myocardial infarction. There is no intention to belittle or denigrate the necessity of knowledge and expertise regarding the physiology and pathology of myocardial infarction and the physical or practical care given to patients who have had a myocardial infarction. The review is structured around three facets of the nursing care of a patient following myocardial infarction that were identifiable in all the suggested regimes of care that were considered, namely, rest, relief of pain and rehabilitation.

Rest has been seen by many writers as an essential influence on successful recovery following myocardial infarction (e.g., Chilman and Thomas, 1981; Read *et al.*, 1984). Despite a rapid change over the past 10 years from a 3–4 week period of bed rest to 24 hours rest followed by gradual mobilisation, emphasis is still placed on restriction and often regimented regimes of graduated activity which add little to an aim of individualised care, claim Farrel *et al.* (1985). They go on to suggest that the best person to decide on activity is the patient, within broad overall schemes suggested by nursing staff.

It could be argued that patients attempting to deny illness might over-exert themselves but if careful assessment of psychological factors is undertaken, as advocated by Thomas (1982), this type of potential problem will almost certainly be revealed.

Wilson-Barnett and Fordham (1982) claim that the fashion for bed rest and restriction of activity has passed its heyday not only because of potential physiological problems such as pressure sores, pneumonia, decalcification of bones and deep venous thrombosis but also because of its detrimental psychological effects leading to malaise, depression and apathy.

The suggestion then is not that rest is unnecessary but that a physiological approach to its achievement such as restriction of activity does not achieve what Read *et al.* (1984) define as 'mental tranquility' or true rest.

Wallace *et al.* (1982) assert that their research supports the view that the use of relaxation training can make a critical contribution to prognosis following a myocardial infarction. This is reiterated by Ward (1983) who also identifies a link between psychological disturbances, such as distress, and sudden death due to arrhythmias.

Pain has been seen as a cardinal feature of myocardial infarction (Houston and White, 1985), and its relief is often identified as the most important aspect of caring for a patient following a myocardial infarction. Thomas (1982) promotes the use of opiates not only to reduce pain but also because of their useful effect on fear and distress, thus decreasing the release of catecholamines and the resultant risk of arrhythmias. The profound psychological effects of pain have been identified by Hilgard *et al.* (1979) as including depression, apathy and fear. It could be argued that pain does not have a totally direct effect on physiology but its effect is mediated by its psychological consequences. Gooch (1984) has written of the major effect of psychological factors both on the physiological consequences of injury and the perception of pain. Gooch's work is mainly related to surgery but may have implications for pain relief following myocardial infarction. The premise is that use of strategies such as giving information, explanation and support will reduce the need for analgesia without compromising effective pain relief. Much research evidence is quoted by Gooch (1984) to support her views.

The restoration of the patient to as 'normal' a life-style as possible following recovery from myocardial infarction is promoted as a general aim of patient care by Chilman and Thomas (1981). No definition of 'normal' is given but the inference is that it means 'as before the infarction'.

The factors determining the success of rehabilitation have been explored by Wilson-Barnett and Fordham (1982). They quote the research of Croog *et al.* (1968) who found that family and social support were major determinants of successful rehabilitation and that return to work was influenced more by occupational and employment opportunities than by patient motivation. They link return to work with social class rather than physiological ability to work.

Depression has been seen as a feature of patients' psychological state following myocardial infarction and as a stumbling block on the path to rehabilitation (McGurn, 1981). Thus social and psychological factors are major influences on patients' return to a 'normal' life-style.

The role of nurses as educators is promoted by Thomas (1982) and Ward (1983). This is another example of the perceived way in which non-physical care has a major influence on the outcome of myocardial infarction. Naismith *et al.* (1979) found pre-discharge counselling had a significant influence on patients' return to work, their physical and emotional stability and their social independence.

In summary, Wilson-Barnett and Fordham (1982) present a closely argued case to support their final assertion that 'most of the care needed for these patients is psychological – their fears being the main source of impaired recovery'. The same may also be said of Gooch (1984) who presents reasoned arguments to support her views. It may be a generalisation but writers promoting strategies of nursing care based on psychological and sociological perspectives appear to be more inclined or able to support their views with logic and research in comparison to writers heavily based in physiological considerations who sometimes tend to produce their views as dogma, unsupported by logic or research evidence.

Justification for choice of model

Collister (1986) has written of the need for a chosen model to accord with the nurse's personal philosophy and view of nursing. The writer of this chapter finds the concentration of Peplau's model on communication, mutual development and an interactionist approach to nurse–patient relationships very much in accord with his own views.

However Aggleton and Chalmers (1985) warn against an unreasoned, intuitive basis to this choice and argue that it is important to consider the appropriateness of the model for understanding the particular patient and his needs.

It has been argued that non-physiological aspects of care are essential considerations when organising the nursing care of patients after myocardial infarction. Use of systems models with a strong biological basis may be seen as promoting an approach to care that is weighted towards physiological concerns although this may not exclude psychological and social considerations. For this reason, the model generally in use on the ward (Henderson's model) was thought not to be ideal for the organisation of Mr Fletcher's care.

Peplau's model evolved from a theory of interpersonal relations in nursing based on psychoanalytical theory (Meleis, 1985). Peplau's basic commitment is to interactionist theory with its implications of negotiated roles and relationships (Meleis, 1985). Thus not only are psychological and social considerations brought sharply into focus, with emphasis on the nurse's roles as teacher, communicator and counsellor (Fitzpatrick and Whall, 1983) rather than bed-bather, drug administrator or monitor-watcher but also the patient is enabled to become an equal partner in determining the care he receives – something seen as desirable by Kratz (1979).

This different emphasis begs the criticism that, firstly, the patient's physical or practical care may be neglected, and secondly, the emphasis on negotiation and patient control may result in totally inappropriate care, for example, heavy strenuous exercise the day after infarction. Both these possible problems are negated by Peplau's emphasis on the nurse as a 'health care professional'. The nurse accepts established knowledge about nursing practice with the proviso that it is critically examined (Fitzpatrick and Whall, 1983). Thus the risk of undisciplined freedom causing neglect or damage is negated by the maintenance of accepted standards (though these are certainly not blindly adhered to).

The word anxiety is often used to describe the feeling of tension and fear following a myocardial infarction. Indeed it is sometimes used as a blanket term to cover all the negative psychological effects of hospitalisation and illness (Chilman and Thomas, 1981; Cook, 1983). Peplau addresses directly the concept of anxiety in what would appear to be a more specific way than any other nursing model. It is precisely defined and, except in limited circumstances, it is not viewed as a problem but rather as the useful and natural tension resulting from a difficulty and creating the energy or arousal necessary to achieve solution of difficulties (Riehl and Roy, 1980). Thus, what has been vaguely defined as a central problem following infarction is one of the primary concerns of this model.

The choice of model, therefore, was made on the basis of the possibility of it enabling a higher standard of care for Mr Fletcher than any other. It focuses on the psychological aspects of care that have been seen as the ones most important following myocardial infarction (Wilson-Barnett and Fordham, 1982) but remains firmly grounded in accepted nursing practice.

Description and utilisation of the model

Peplau views a human being as an organism living in unstable equilibrium with the environment. This situation results in needs or deviations from the desired state. The tension (often recognised as anxiety) created by these needs provides the energy for learning and problem-solving behaviours (Riehl and Roy, 1980).

The ability to learn and solve problems is seen as central to a continuous development and maturation which is essential to human nature (Fitzpatrick and Whall, 1983). This view of the need for

development by a process of meeting needs is congruent with that of Maslow, who proposed a hierarchy of needs with individuals satisfying each level before progressing to 'higher things', with the ultimate goal of 'self-actualisation' as the pinnacle of achievement (Hilgard *et al.*, 1979).

Peplau considers nursing as a therapeutic interpersonal process that aids patients both to gain intellectual and interpersonal competencies beyond those which they have at the point of illness and to progress from the less mature developmental stages that predominate during illness (Fitzpatrick and Whall, 1983). It may be possible to support the view of illness causing regression to less mature states by use of the arguments of Parsons regarding the 'sick-role' and his claim that a person who becomes sick feels able to abrogate responsibilities and behaviours that are concomitant with adulthood (Patrick and Scambler, 1982).

Peplau's commitment to interactionism is not only reflected in her view of the nurse–patient relationship as an open fluid entity with a commitment to equal status and control. She also identifies various roles adopted by or required of the nurse at different stages of the relationship – stranger, resource, teacher, leader, surrogate, counsellor (Fitzpatrick and Whall, 1983).

Peplau views the nurse's maturity and ability to integrate a variety of experiences as essential to effective nursing (Fitzpatrick and Whall, 1983). What the patient learns during nursing depends on the kind of person the nurse is (Riehl and Roy, 1980). It is not only the patient who develops as a result of the provision of nursing; the nurse also undergoes maturation and experiences learning (Riehl and Roy, 1980).

Integration of Peplau's model with the nursing process

Peplau's model is not structured with reference to the nursing process. However, she writes of four stages of nursing – orientation, identification, exploitation and resolution. These stages have been seen as parallel with the four stages of the nursing process (Riehl and Roy, 1980).

Orientation/assessment

Peplau defines orientation as the beginning of the nurse–patient relationship. The patient is willing to accept help and is attempting to learn the nature of present difficulties and the assistance required. The patient may be tense and nervous but this is seen as productive because of the energy arousal it produces. Peplau argues that needs should be mutually agreed between nurse and patient but, if a need is perceived by the nurse as an emergency that cannot be left until agreement is reached, it can be acted upon (Riehl and Roy, 1980).

Peplau has used the word 'stranger' to describe the role of the nurse at the beginning of orientation. The qualities she sees as facets of the role include courtesy, respect, positive interest and non-judgemental acceptance (Fitzpatrick and Whall, 1983). She promotes a gradual formation of the nurse–patient relationship rather than the immediate assumption of a stereotyped relationship where the nurse, despite 'a polite appearance of consensus', is firmly in control (Rosenthal *et al.*, 1980).

The elements of orientation are directly transferable to assessment using Peplau's model. Both Peplau and Kratz (1979) would see the end result of assessment as a list of patient-validated problems that are jointly discovered and agreed.

What then constitutes a problem when using Peplau's model? Riehl and Roy (1980) define it as 'the originating point of deviation from the desired state or condition'. Examples might be a person unable to tie a shoelace following a cerebral vascular accident, an adolescent unable to form friendships or loss of continence following a prostatectomy. Problems are not always so overt or apparent to the patient. This is one area where the nurse contributes knowledge and expertise in the role of resource, teacher or leader – but not dictator (Fitzpatrick and Whall, 1983).

As well as mutual identification of problems by a process of logical thought and discussion, it may be possible to identify a difficulty or need by first discovering anxiety and tension. Peplau claims these feelings arise directly as a result of deviation

from the desired state (Meleis, 1985). An example might be a patient anxious about getting out of bed and walking to the lavatory. The underlying problem might be poor balance, transient dizziness, impaired vision or urgency of micturition – once anxiety is identified as arising from the situation or activity then further analysis may reveal the problem.

It might be possible to construct a questionnaire-type assessment form based on the basic concerns of Peplau's model but this would place constraints on free interaction and, by the nature of printed sheets, would impose a prioritisation of areas for discussion by differing allocation of space and order. The assessment for this care plan was carried out using a blank sheet of paper but, because of a lack of familiarity with non-structured assessment, the writer prepared a list of possible questions to guide the conversation if it appeared to flag or go off at a tangent. The questions were all concerned with aspects of the model such as tension, anxiety, roles, communication, relationships and deviations from desired states (Fig. 6.1).

It would be difficult to note everything said in conversations of this type. The recording of points mutually agreed to be significant and questions used to redirect conversation was thought sufficient.

Identification/planning

Peplau sees the next stage of the nurse–patient relationship as being characterised by the patient's identification with the nurse and vice versa. The quality of empathy comes to the fore with the nurse attempting to view the identified problems through the patient's eyes and the patient understanding the nurse's perspective and appreciating the information and advice that is offered (Riehl and Roy, 1980).

Identification and growing closer might well occur during the assessment process and some of the planning stage might involve further orientation. However, Riehl and Roy (1980) see identification as concurrent with planning – the joint formulation of a care plan being a major contribution to this drawing together.

Fig. 6.1 Assessment

> *Do you have any particular worries at present?*
>
> Concerned at how others will cope while he is in hospital. Has letters to write and people to see.
>
> Concerned that his present condition is related to previous endocarditis.
>
> Sees heart attack as a warning to slow down but afraid his son will not respect him if he regards him as an invalid.
>
> Knows that diet can be important in heart disease but has no idea what he should or should not eat.
>
> Feels weak but does not want to become bedbound.
>
> *Does anything worry you about having a heart attack?*
>
> Not afraid of dying – 'it comes to us all'.
>
> Afraid of the dreadful pain coming back.
>
> Wants to know how to avoid complications that may follow a heart attack.
>
> Hates using commode at bed side (as happened in CCU).
>
> *How do you feel about transferring to the ward from CCU?*
>
> Told it is a step towards discharge, so pleased.
>
> Feeling a bit worried about leaving high technology, high expertise area.
>
> Hopes it may mean less time in bed (nursed in bed in CCU)
>
> Looking forward to having more people to talk to – did not realise he would be in a side ward.
>
> *What do you think the heart attack will stop you doing?*
>
> Will stop playing golf and tennis but hopes to continue walking as a pastime.
>
> Will mean reducing responsibilities to social groups and other organisations.
>
> Will give up work even though he enjoys it. Hopes his wife will understand his need to 'slow down'.
>
> *What information do you feel you need?*
>
> What he can do to get better quicker.
>
> What activities he can continue when he is discharged.
>
> Dietary advice.
>
> What the ward routine is.
>
> *Anything else you wish to say?*
>
> Knows his elder son will cope well with his illness but very unsure about his younger son who hates weakness or ill health.

When preparing the goals that will represent the solution or alleviation of the listed problems it must first be established why intervention is being planned (Fig. 6.2). For example, anxiety is an indication in its own right: the goal 'to reduce expressed anxiety' might be viewed as a recommendation to treat the symptom rather than the cause and would not be compatible with Peplau's model.

However, 'deviation from the desired state or condition' may be alleviated in two ways. Firstly by enabling the patient to achieve the desired state or condition. Secondly, by promoting an understanding and resignation to the impossibility of achieving it. Either solution results in the diminishing of anxiety and this may be a useful measure of success.

Exploitation/implementation

Exploitation is characterised by the patient making full use of the interventions decided upon during the identification/planning stage both in the sense of physical care and the other roles of the nurse such as counsellor, teacher, leader, surrogate, and resource. The interventions or strategies that are agreed upon and implemented during this stage depend on what the patient views as useful and the nurse's ability to produce a range of alternatives – again, professional knowledge is necessary (Meleis, 1985).

Implementation of care using Peplau's model involves as much talking and listening as it does performing physical tasks (Meleis, 1985). This reflects a change of emphasis from the traditional role of the nurse but is clearly supported in the literature already cited. It would appear that in many situations, psychological and social factors have more influence on the success of a period of hospitalisation, from the patient's point of view, than physical care (Patrick and Scambler, 1982).

Resolution/evaluation

During the resolution phase of the evolving nurse–patient relationship, old ties and dependencies may be relinquished and an evaluation is made of the growth and maturation undergone by both

Fig. 6.2   Care plan

Problem, need or difficulty	Goal	Intervention	Evaluation	Date
Day 1 Unable to relax and forget his commitments. Feels he's let down the various social groups and organisations he belongs to.	Will feel that he's done as much as he can given his present situation and will express a cessation of his feelings of guilt.	1 Helped to make list of his commitments. 2 Encouraged to ring up two friends who belong to same groups as him and can take over his commitments. 3 Reinforcement given of his own belief that he needs to be a little selfish at this stage of his life. 4 Suggestion made that he should ask his wife to write letters to the chairmen and other chief organisers of the groups he belongs to acquainting them with his indisposition.	Volunteered information that he feels everything needed has been done and feels a weight off his shoulders. Very positive reactions from the groups he belongs to. Floods of 'get well' cards and flowers.	Day 4
Feels he should know about complications of heart attack and how to detect and avoid them.	Will express confidence in his knowledge without becoming obsessional and introspective.	1 Simple explanations given and repeated of what a heart attack is, what the most common complications are, how they manifest themselves, their treatment and avoidance. 2 Physiotherapist involved to teach deep breathing and circulation improving exercises. 3 Taught how to keep a fluid balance chart and encouraged to maintain it himself.	Feels he knows more about how his body works and especially about the possible complications following a heart attack.	Day 9

Fig. 6.2 (continued)

Problem, need or difficulty	Goal	Intervention	Evaluation	Date
Feels weary and knows he should take it easy but hates to be inactive.	Will not cause strain on the heart by mobilising too quickly but will retain control over his own level of activity.	1 Shown ward standard regime for mobilisation following myocardial infarction and encouraged to decide on what he feels able to do each day and not to exceed this. 2 Mrs Fletcher encouraged to bring in tapes and books to help ward off boredom.	No intervention required to limit Mr Fletcher's mobility or activity. Is now fully mobile about ward area and hospital grounds with no negative consequences.	Day 7
Dissatisfied with his knowledge about the diet recommended.	Will choose a high-fibre, low polyunsaturated fat diet when filling in menu cards. Will express confidence in his ability to choose a suitable diet.	1 Dietician asked to see Mr Fletcher and his wife. Given spoken and written information about diet and ischaemic heart disease. 2 Initially helped to identify high-fibre, low polyunsaturated fat food on menu cards.	Ordering high-fibre, low polyunsaturated fat diet without assistance. Asked how confident he felt about his ability – just a smug expression!	
Worried about how he'd cope with recurrence of his chest pain.	Will express diminished anxiety about pain. Will understand the different types of pain that follow a myocardial infarction and the way they may be dealt with.	1 Informed that although he may get chest pain at this stage it will not be as severe as during the acute phase of infarction. 2 Shown drug sheet and advised that any pain will be adequately treated but he will have to tell us he's got it.	Except one minor attack (of angina) that responded to glyceryl trinitrate no severe chest pain.	Day 9

Fig. 6.2   (continued)

Problem, need or difficulty	Goal	Intervention	Evaluation	Date
Day 3 Unsure how his son will react to his illness and how it will affect their relationship.	Will know how his son feels and accept any change in their relationship.	1 Suggested that he phone his son and share his fears concerning their relationship. 2 Advised to stop thinking of himself as an invalid and that he'd be able to return to his previous life-style minus the activities that he identified as stressful.	Son sent long letter expressing his love. Mr Fletcher felt he wished to share his letter with me. Son also enclosed set of British Heart Foundation leaflets.	Day 5
Day 9 Concerned about what he should be doing at home after discharge.	Will leave the ward expressing confidence in his knowledge about post-discharge activity.	1 Given spoken and written advice about resumption of work, golf, driving, sex, etc. 2 Given ward telephone number and encouraged to phone if he had any problems.	Left ward expressing more confidence about activities but told staff to expect him to ring if he had any worries.	Day 9

patient and nurse. Some writers (e.g., Riehl and Roy, 1980) claim that Peplau views this evaluation as being carried out by the nurse alone but this would seem contrary to the interactionist nature of the model, which would suggest a joint evaluative process.

The evaluation stage of the nursing process leads to a recycling of the process and this is not reflected in the concept of relinquishing a relationship. Instead, it appears more congruent with summative evaluation or audit as advocated by Kratz (1979). Peplau's model envisages nursing promoting growth and maturation – such an outcome will be greater than the parts of problems solved.

To evaluate the benefits of using this model to organise his care, Mr Fletcher's opinion was sought. It could be argued that Mr Fletcher's situation precluded his criticism or expression of dissatisfaction with the care he had been offered because of his reluctance to offend or because of his perceived vulnerability as a patient dependent on health carers. Because of the relationship developed, the writer of this chapter believes that Mr Fletcher's views were honest and complete. To negate the second possible influence on his willingness to criticise the evaluation took place only an hour before Mr Fletcher was discharged, with him dressed and his belongings packed, in an office away from the ward environment. His comments and remarks are presented in Fig. 6.3 of this chapter and form the bulk of the evaluation of the use of this model.

Critique of Peplau's model

Peplau's model has been criticised on several grounds. Fitzpatrick and Whall (1983) suggest that

Fig. 6.3 Evaluation by Mr Fletcher

> Feels that nursing staff on the wards have been friends rather than people to look after him.
>
> The most important contribution by the nurses was their support and guidance which helped him through the experience of having a heart attack. Feels this has improved his prospects of returning to a normal life.
>
> Being encouraged to make his own decisions helped him to retain his independence and identity. Even small things like choosing his own food and deciding when he was able to have a shower were important.
>
> Felt safe.
>
> Has learned that he has been doing too much and that there need to be some changes in his life. Has learned the value of coping with distractions and interruptions without becoming tense and angry. Feels that his relationship with his younger son is more secure. Feels family members are more open about their love for each other.
>
> Feels he is more aware of his own mortality and the need to live life to the full without the burden of too many responsibilities.
>
> Feels he can enjoy membership of social groups without taking on major organisational roles.
>
> *Is there anything you think you have learned on the ward?*
>
> Knows more about his body and especially the functioning of his heart.
>
> Feels he and his wife know more about suitable foods.
>
> Feels he has learned a lot about his own feelings and those of his family.
>
> Feels the care plan provided a useful summary of the things that worried him.

Peplau promotes the concept of unlimited growth with an emphasis on increasingly mature goals similar to that of Maslow (Hilgard *et al.*, 1979). They see this as overly idealistic and the source of much possible frustration and dissatisfaction, but to place a ceiling on possible growth might be viewed as restrictive rather than realistic. They suggest that Peplau concentrates on illness to the exclusion of consideration of healthy individuals but this seems somewhat over-critical if one considers that Peplau is writing about the care of patients and makes no claim to a detailed analysis of other relationships.

The concentration of Peplau's model on the relationship between two individuals may appear alien to the situation on some wards where shift systems separate nurse and patient for days on end. Two solutions might be offered for this discrepancy. Primary nursing could facilitate the role of one nurse in establishing the care plan for a patient and being responsible for updating this plan. The extra communication and continuity of care made possible by the nursing process (Kratz, 1979) might allow the relationship to be between the patient and a team or group of nurses.

If the idea of a one-to-one relationship as the basis for 'good' care is to be accepted, then the central role of this relationship within nursing settings is crucial. Further careful use of the model is needed to try to establish what outcomes might occur if the nurse–patient relationship does not prove to be productive. A model of care that emphasises the building of relationships rather than the completion of physical tasks will require not only different nursing skills but also an awareness of the range of potential outcomes.

Evaluation of the model in use

Evaluation was carried out (Fig. 6.3) and is presented in a similar way to assessment. A blank sheet of paper was used to record Mr Fletcher's opinions in note form and this was checked and validated by him. Also recorded is a question that may have influenced his answers or changed the direction of the discussion. The inclusion of the writer's opinions and feelings was considered but rejected as overly subjective and possibly biased. Suffice it to say that this implementation was not only educative and of benefit to standards of care on the ward but was also an enjoyable and emotionally rewarding experience.

References

Aggleton P & Chalmers H 1985 Models and theories. *Nursing Times*, April 3: 36–39.
Chilman AM & Thomas M 1981 *Understanding Nursing Care*. Churchill Livingstone, Edinburgh.

Collister B   1986   Psychiatric nursing and a developmental model. In *Models for Nursing*, B Kershaw & J Savage (Eds). John Wiley & Sons, Chichester.

Cook J   1983   Myocardial infarction. *Nursing Mirror*, May 11: iii–iv.

Croog SH, Levine S & Lurie Z   1968   The heart patient and the recovery process. *Social Science and Medicine*, 2: 111–164.

Farrel J, Booth E & Hayburne T   1985   Telling it straight. *Nursing Mirror*, 1 May: 51–52.

Fitzpatrick JJ & Whall AL (Eds)   1983   *Conceptual Models of Nursing: Analysis and Application*. Robert J Brady Co, Maryland.

Gooch J   1984   *The Other Side of Surgery*. Macmillan, London.

Henderson V   1966   *The Nature of Nursing: A definition and its implications, practice, research and education*. Macmillan, New York.

Hilgard ER, Atkinson RC & Atkinson RL   1979   *Introduction to Psychology*. New York, Harcourt Brace Jovanovich.

Houston JC & White HH   1985   *Principles of Medicine and Medical Nursing*. Hodder & Stoughton, London.

Kratz CR   1979   *The Nursing Process*. Baillière Tindall, London.

McGurn WC   1981   *People with Cardiac Problems*. Lippincott, London.

Meleis AI   1985   *Theoretical Nursing*. Lippincott, Philadelphia.

Naismith LD, Robinson JF, Shaw GB & MacIntyre MMJ   1979   Psychological rehabilitation after myocardial infarction. *British Medical Journal*, i: 439–446.

Patrick DL & Scambler G   1982   *Sociology as Applied to Medicine*. Baillière Tindall, London.

Read AE, Barritt DW & Langton Hewer R   1984   *Modern Medicine*. Pitman, London.

Riehl JP & Roy C (Eds)   1980   *Conceptual Models for Nursing Practice*. Appleton-Century-Crofts, Norwalk.

Rosenthal CJ, Marshal VW, MacPherson AJ & French SE   1980   *Nursing, Patients and Families*. Croom Helm, London.

Thomas DR   1982   *Cardiac Nursing*. Baillière Tindall, London.

Wallace LM, Bratt-Wyton R, Jones R & Wingett C   1982   Relaxation for heart patients. *Nursing Times*, September 29: 1642–1643.

Ward T   1983   Coronary care. *Nursing Mirror*, May 11: i–ii.

Wilson-Barnett J & Fordham M   1982   *Recovery from Illness*. John Wiley & Sons, Chichester.

7

Care plan for a woman with cardiac failure, using Roper's Activities of Living model

Anne Chew and Anne PM Williams

Introduction

The neighbourhood hospital in which this study of care took place has 40 beds in which the medical cover is provided by local GPs. The ward consists of two single rooms and an eight-bedded Nightingale-style ward for female patients. There exists a close relationship with social workers, district nurses, GPs and local clergy. Relations and friends have easy access to the hospital which is well known to most patients as it forms an integral part of the community of a small market town. There is a high ratio of nursing auxiliaries to trained nurses on the ward, and no learners. Currently the nursing process is implemented using Henderson's model (Henderson, 1966) but for this particular patient Roper's model (Roper, Logan and Tierney, 1985) was used.

The patient, who likes to be called Annie, is a 77-year-old unmarried woman living locally with her widowed sister. They enjoy an active social life although since 1983 the patient has been restricted by shortness of breath following a deep vein thrombosis and pulmonary embolus. On this present occasion, she was admitted with a history of increasing breathlessness of two weeks' duration. The GP had diagnosed cardiac failure.

On admission an ECG showed an old but previously unsuspected anterior myocardial infarction thought to be responsible for the myocardial insufficiency and breathlessness.

Reasons for using Roper's model of nursing

The hospital has introduced the nursing process using Virginia Henderson's model of nursing. Henderson's model (Henderson, 1966) has been fairly rigidly applied and it was felt a model with a slightly different emphasis would give staff the opportunity to work with new ideas and to be aware of the use of another model. However it was realised that introducing a model based on totally different concepts might cause confusion and opposition in staff who had only recently accepted and implemented Henderson's model. Roper's model (Roper *et al.*, 1985) is based on 'activities of living' which are not dissimilar to Henderson's 'basic needs'. It is a systems model which organises nursing intervention in a fairly traditional way, thus enabling both staff and patients to identify readily with its implementation and aims. On admission it was evident that the patient chosen for this study was cooperative, traditional in her expectations of hospitals and, barring unexpected events, seemed destined to make sufficient improvement to return home and lead a fairly independent life. As the patient's problems were essentially physical, Roper's model of nursing seemed to offer a means of identifying appropriate ways of assisting her. The patient's ultimate aim was to feel physically able to resume her life at home with her sister. It was felt that by using Roper's model of nursing a high standard of relevant care could be delivered to the patient.

It was felt that as many of the models of nursing recently published originated in USA it would be desirable to use one derived from work carried out in British hospitals. Roper's model is now used in a number of NHS hospitals throughout the country and accounts of its implementation are to be found in the nursing literature. Of particular note are the work of the Burford Unit and the books and articles published by Roper, Logan and Tierney. It was found useful to have access to other people's experiences with Roper's model not only in deciding whether it would be a suitable model for the patient but also in planning appropriate nursing interventions and in the use of nursing documentation.

Usefulness of available literature

Literature on Roper's model and its implementation is fairly widely available in books and journals but recent information specifically about the nursing care of a patient with cardiac failure can only be found in standard nursing textbooks.

Cardiac failure occurs when the heart cannot maintain sufficient blood supply for the body tissues. In Annie's case the myocardial insufficiency was due to damage to the heart muscle from an old anterior myocardial infarction. According to Herbert (1984) common symptoms associated with cardiac failure include oedema, cyanosis, dyspnoea, loss of appetite, indigestion and constipation. For Annie, however, the major problem was one of acute breathlessness. Intervention therefore was likely to focus on improving cardiac efficiency, facilitating breathing and preventing undue oxygen demands being made by the body.

Kitchen (1984) describes the physiology of heart failure, its consequences and the types of drug therapy commonly in use. He describes how digoxin therapy improves cardiac output and diuretics reduce the blood volume thus improving the efficiency of the heart.

Major problems with heart failure are discussed by Cooke (1982) who stresses that goals set to increase mobility and independence should reflect the ability of the heart to cope with increasing work load. Wilson-Barnett (1986) discusses problems experienced by a 72-year-old person with a medical diagnosis of heart failure and appears to use a nursing framework similar to that of Roper. Breathlessness is recognised as being a major problem and nursing intervention is designed to reduce the oxygen requirements of the body. In accordance with Cooke (1982), Wilson-Barnett (1986) emphasises that the patient's own energy levels are critical in planning activities and goals. Durie (1984) describes the nursing management of people with a range of common respiratory problems. Here also, interventions aim to conserve energy, administer prescribed medical treatments and relieve the anxiety so often accompanying breathlessness. Durie (1984) also provides useful ideas for teaching someone to cope with chronic respiratory problems, such as how to pace their activities and how to carry out exercises to improve their breathing.

The model

The model of nursing known as Roper's model first appeared in 1980 in *The Elements of Nursing*, the work of Roper, Logan and Tierney. It was based on a model developed by Roper from research carried out in Britain between 1970 and 1974. Roper's model has continued to be refined and modified as currently presented in a second edition of *The Elements of Nursing* (1985).

The focus of this model is on 12 activities of living (AL) which have relevance for everyone. In carrying out each AL an individual may be dependent on others to a variable degree. This continuum of dependency is affected by a wide range of factors. One factor singled out for special consideration is age since a person's capacity for independence alters with the stages of their life span. For example a newborn baby breathes independently but is totally dependent for its nutritional needs. At the other end of the life span an elderly person may be able to feed independently but require assistance with mobility.

The activities of living identified by Roper are:

1   maintaining a safe environment;
2   communicating;
3   breathing;

4 eating and drinking;
5 eliminating;
6 personal cleansing and dressing;
7 controlling body temperature;
8 mobilising;
9 working and playing;
10 expressing sexuality;
11 sleeping;
12 dying.

Each of these ALs has biological, developmental and social components. For example, the activity of communicating is highly complex. If we consider verbal communication, certain physical characteristics are necessary in order that vocal sounds can be made. In addition the skills of language use develop both as a result of age and as a result of social interaction.

Roper, Logan and Tierney based their model of nursing on a model of living, and nursing is seen as assisting people prevent, solve or alleviate problems related to their ALs. People may experience actual problems or may have potential problems. When these are identified nursing intervention may take place to solve or alleviate the actual problems or to prevent potential problems becoming actual problems.

Roper, Logan and Tierney (1985) state that individualised nursing is necessary due to individuality in living and, as most people require nursing only for short periods during their life, it should not disrupt their life-style more than necessary. To accomplish individualised nursing care it is essential therefore to know about the patient's individuality in living. This may be achieved by assessing each activity of living with that patient and identifying actual or potential problems related to them. A nursing plan related to the ALs can then be devised by setting goals and selecting interventions specifically related to the ALs and the achievement of these goals.

Roper's model and the nursing process

During assessment the activities performed independently are recorded as well as those which require assistance. Those ALs which cannot be carried out independently are treated as problems. Physical, social and psychological perspectives are considered and the patient's usual routine is ascertained.

Thus, following assessment of the ALs, actual and potential problems are identified. In consultation with the patient, goals are set and nursing intervention planned to try to achieve these goals. Long-term goals are likely to aim for independence in ALs or for acceptance of any necessary dependence. Roper's model acknowledges the need for some nursing interventions to be organised around medical prescription which may not be related directly to activities of living. Such interventions may include drug administration and could be incorporated in the nursing care plan. Roper, Logan and Tierney (1985), however, suggest documenting such intervention separately.

Nursing intervention centres on the fulfilment of the ALs and may involve providing comfort, protection and assistance. Maintaining a life-style as similar to the patient's usual one as possible reduces anxiety and confusion and facilitates return to independent living.

Assessment of the effectiveness of nursing intervention is the aim of evaluation. Achievement of goals is one measure of success but other changes are difficult to quantify. Reassessment may be required to determine whether the goals were realistic and appropriate and whether the nursing intervention was effective and suitable.

Evaluation of use of model

In evaluating the Roper model of nursing consideration will be given to the documentation used, the four parts of the nursing process – assessment, planning, intervention, evaluation – and to the overall value of the model and reactions to its use by other staff.

The documentation used is similar to that used by Stewart and Strachen (1983). The biographical data includes information such as that outlined by the Patient Assessment Form (Roper *et al.*, 1981) together with additions such as past nursing history which we felt might identify relevant information (for example, a previous unhappy experience in hospital), space for writing recordings made on admission – temperature, pulse, respirations and urinalysis, a check list for discharge preparations and space for recording medically prescribed tests such as ECGs and blood investigations. The form

used for assessment (Fig. 7.1) was left blank as far as possible to allow for flexibility when assessing each AL. Thus restrictions were not present in terms of space which might influence the quality and quantity of data recorded.

Each problem identified was recorded in the

Fig. 7.1 Assessment

Usual routine: *what patient can/cannot do independently*			
Activities of living	**Date**	**Assessment of activities of living**	**Patient's problem** (A = actual, P = potential)
Maintaining a safe environment	28.7	Walks with 2 sticks due to osteoarthritis in hips. Sits on stool in bath since fall in bath 6 months ago. Has stairs – manages if she takes it slowly. Knows own limitations and aware of potential dangers.	P *Risk of falling* due to limited mobility and changed environment.
Communicating	28.7	Coherent, fluent speech. Breathless after talking for short length of time. No hearing difficulties. Wears glasses for reading. Is fully orientated. Visits friends and receives regular visitors at home. Married sister lives next door – has car and will visit daily together with sister who lives with Annie.	
Breathing	28.7	Says she is always breathless if pursuing any activity for long before sitting down. Wakes short of breath at night – after slipping down in bed. Does not smoke. Has been more breathless over past 2 weeks since returning from holiday. On Admission – breathless at rest. Lips cyanosed. Extremities not cyanosed. No ankle oedema. Pulse is regularly irregular – 70 per min. Resps – 28 per min. BP 150/90. No cough. Says she is not anxious about her breathlessness as 'used to it'.	A *Breathless at rest and on slightest exertion.*
	28.7	Following discussion, Annie's sister confirms she becomes breathless on any exertion – talking, washing, walking etc. Some days are worse than others. Breathlessness worse recently.	
Eating and drinking	28.7	Enjoys food though 'not a big eater'. Avoids fried foods, likes fruit and vegetables. Has main meal at midday. Drinks about 8 glasses of fluid daily. Sister does the shopping. Annie and sister share cooking.	
Eliminating	28.7	Bowels open regularly every 3–4 days for soft stool – normal for Annie. Passes urine once during night – uses commode. No pain, burning or incontinence. Takes diuretics therefore passes urine more in mornings. Has downstairs and upstairs toilet.	

Fig. 7.1 (continued)

Usual routine: *what patient can/cannot do independently*			
Activities of living	**Date**	**Assessment of activities of living**	**Patient's problem** (A = actual, P = potential)
Personal cleansing and dressing	28.7	Dresses independently – needs occasional help from sister with stockings. Baths once a week using bath stool. Sister helps get in and out. Has strip wash at sink alternate days or as needed. Has dentures which she leaves in at night. Visits hairdresser once a week.	A *Difficulty with washing while confined to bed and whilst experiencing increased breathlessness.*
Controlling body temperature	28.7	Apyrexial on admission. Has occasional night sweats. Leaves window open at night. House has central heating.	
Mobilising	28.7	Walks with 2 sticks. Has slight stoop. Wears corset since fractured vertebrae from fall 6 months ago. Has pain in knees on walking due to osteoarthritis. Gets breathless after walking a few feet. Uses wheelchair outside home. Raises self independently from chair, bed and toilet. In bed for last two days since increased shortness of breath.	P *Increased stiffness and immobility.* P *Increased joint pain* since non steroidal anti-inflammatory drug stopped. P *Risk of deep vein thrombosis* – previous pulmonary embolus. P *Risk of pressure sores.*
Working and playing	28.7	Hobbies include gardening – uses dutch hoe. Watches TV. Goes out for trips in sister's car. Recently returned from 2 week holiday in Bournemouth. Gets breathless if active. 'Knows when to stop.' Used to work as a nursing auxiliary.	
Expressing sexuality	28.7	Does not regret being single. Takes interest in nieces and nephews. Not embarrassed about using commode.	
Sleeping	28.7	Normally retires to bed 11 pm wakes 9 am. Does not mind sleeping in ward with other patients. Always wakes between 2 am and 3 am and awake for approximately 1 hour. Wants to take sleeping tablets if possible (does not usually take them).	P *Disturbed sleep.*
Dying	28.7	Not worried at prospect of dying 'I've seen so much of it', but does not feel ill enough to die.	

nursing care plan together with goals set. Planned interventions were written, with a rationale for the choice of intervention made and a date for evaluation was noted (Fig. 7.2).

A written record of progress, related specifically to goal evaluation, was found to be useful. Modifications to the care plan were also a feature of this evaluation sheet (Fig 7.3).

Most of the ALs were assessed at interview on the day of admission. As the AL of breathing was seen as a priority this was assessed first and other ALs were assessed later when Annie was less breathless. All the ALs were assessed as it became apparent that many were interrelated and, as Aggleton and Chalmers (1985) argue, some assessment of each activity is necessary to ensure no actual or potential problems are ignored.

The Roper model, in identifying activities of

Fig. 7.2   Nursing care plan for Miss Annie West

Date	Problem related to AL	Goal	Date	Intervention	Rationale	Evaluation date	Date problem resolved
28.7	*Breathing* A Breathless at rest and on slightest exertion	Patient will: 1 Not be breathless at rest.	28.7	Administer prescribed medication. Continue to nurse in bed in upright position. Record 4-hourly temperature, pulse and apex beat, respiratory rate and record fluid intake and output. Administer oxygen 4 litres per min. via Hudson mask if cyanosed. Assist with washing. Assist to use commode when necessary.	Rest in upright position improves chest expansion and decreases respiratory effort (Cooke, 1982). Recording accurate fluid intake and output helps to monitor affects of diuretic therapy (Wilson-Barnett, 1986). Assisting with activities that may induce shortness of breath helps to reduce cardiac work load – a main aim when caring for patients in heart failure (McGurn, 1981).	Each shift for 24 hours	31.7 Patient no longer breathless at rest.
		2 Not be breathless while talking.				Each shift for 24 hours	
		3 State she is less breathless than prior to admission while performing usual daily activities.		Ask Annie to liaise with sister to reduce number of visitors and length of visiting time.		Daily	2.8 Patient not breathless when talking.
28.7	*Maintaining a safe environment* P Risk of falling	Patient will not fall while in hospital.	28.7	Nurse to assist Annie when she gets into and out of bed.		Report if problem arises.	

Date	Problem/Need	Goal	Date	Nursing action	Rationale		Evaluation
28.7	*Personal washing and dressing* A Difficulty with washing	Patient will: 1 Feel clean and fresh while confined to bed. 2 Be able to wash unaided.	1.8	Provide high chair when sitting. Provide sticks for walking and obstacle free environment. Nurse to accompany when walking. Encourage use of sticks when walking.	Matching chair and bed to suit individual needs assists with maintaining safe environment (Roper et al., 1980).	Daily	31.7 Able to wash unaided.
			29.7	Blanket bath and wash as requested by Annie.			
			30.7	Wash at wash basin sitting down – nurse to assist.			
			31.7	Wash at wash basin unaided. Nurse to assist if breathless.			
28.7	*Mobilising* P Increased stiffness and immobility.	Will continue to perform usual activities of living independently.	31.7	Wash independently at wash basin.		Daily	4.8 Able to perform usual activities.
			1.8	As above. Sit out for 2 hours divided intervals.			
			2.8	As above plus 4 hours in chair. Walk round ward am and pm.			
	P Increased joint pain since discontinuing usual non steroidal anti-inflammatory drug.	Will be pain free at rest and performing usual ALs	28.7	Administer prescribed 4-hourly paracetamol.	Aim of use for analgesic in controlling chronic pain is for regular administration before pain returns (Collins and Parker, 1981).	Daily	4.8 Is pain free.
			1.8	Administer Benoral as prescribed. Ask 4-hourly if in pain and give paracetamol as necessary.			

Fig. 7.2 (continued)

Date	Problem related to AL	Goal	Date	Intervention	Rationale	Evaluation date	Date problem resolved
	P Deep vein thrombosis while confined to bed.	Will not develop deep vein thrombosis as demonstrated by non-swollen pain-free limbs with temperature same as rest of skin.	28.7	Teach and ask patient to perform 2-hourly lower limb movements. Ambulate as above as soon as shortness of breath permits.	Early ambulation increases muscle pump action and reduces homeostasis (Turner and Turner, 1982).	Daily. Record if problem arises.	4.8 No signs of deep vein thrombosis.
	P Pressure sores	Skin will remain intact with no redness or pain at pressure sites.	28.7	Ask patient to change position in bed 2-hourly. Provide sheepskin to lie on in bed. Ambulate as above, as shortness of breath permits.	Relief of pressure by change of position is a fundamental principle in prevention of pressure sores. Use of a sheepskin may help to reduce compression (Roper et al., 1980).	Daily. Record if problem arises. Record if problem arises.	Skin intact.
28.7	*Sleeping* **P** Disturbed sleep	Will sleep for a minimum of 5 consecutive hours each night.	28.7 28.7	Ensure most comfortable position in bed while semi-recumbent to facilitate breathing. Discuss possible use of night sedation with GP.		Daily by night staff. Report if problem arises.	4.8 Is sleeping for more than 5 consecutive hours.

Fig. 7.3 Progress and evaluation record for Miss Annie West

Time and date	Problem		Progress and evaluation	Modification
28.7	A	Shortness of breath	Breathless after talking for prolonged period. Not short of breath at rest. Not cyanosed – has not required oxygen. Respirations 28 per minute. Pulse: 80, Apex: 100. Apyrexial. Seen and examined by GP. Frusemide increased to 120 mg daily. Stat dose of oral frusemide given at 20.00. ECG taken – shows evidence of old anterior myocardial infarction. Blood taken for urea and electrolytes, full blood count and digoxin levels.	
	P	Risk of falling	Able to get in and out of bed to use commode with minimal assistance from nurse. Has not fallen.	
	A	Difficulty in washing	Washed hands and face this evening with bowl provided.	
	P	Increased joint pain	Lederfen discontinued by GP as thought to contribute to fluid retention. Prescribed 4-hourly paracetamol. Patient states she is pain free at rest.	
	P	Deep vein thrombosis (DVT)	Performing 2-hourly leg exercises. No sign of DVT.	
	P	Pressure sores	Pressure areas intact. Turning self 2-hourly in bed.	
29.7	A	Shortness of breath	Good diuresis from frusemide. Not breathless at rest. Less breathless when talking.	
08.00	P	Disturbed sleep	Woke to use commode ×3 but stated she had the best night's sleep for some time. Night sedation prescribed but not given. GP requests avoid if possible.	

Fig. 7.3 (continued)

Time and date	Problem		Progress and evaluation	Modification	
14.00	A	Shortness of breath	Breathless and cyanosed after talking for long period and using commode. Oxygen given intermittently with good effect. Good diuresis maintained.		
	P	Difficulty with washing	Enjoyed blanket bath this morning but would prefer to wash at basin with assistance if shortness of breath allows.	30.7	Wash at basin with assistance.
20.00	A	Shortness of breath	Breathless only when talking for long periods – receiving short visits from family only and allowing them to do most of the talking. Not cyanosed. No oxygen required.		
	P	Risk of falling	Able to get out of bed unaided to use commode.		
	P	Stiffness and immobility	Moving freely in bed. Transferring well from bed to commode.		
	P	Increased joint pain	States paracetamol is controlling pain.		
	P	DVT	No pain or swelling of limbs. Maintaining 2-hourly exercises.		
	P	Pressure sores	Skin remains intact. No redness or pain.		
30.7	A	Shortness of breath	Breathless only after washing hands and face in bed. No cyanosis.		
08.00	P	Disturbed sleep	Woke at 2 am to use commode otherwise slept throughout the night without sedation.		
20.00	A	Shortness of breath	Breathless only on movement now, i.e. washing at basin this morning and transferring from bed to commode. Respirations 24 per minute at rest. Not cyanosed. Remains apyrexial. Seen by GP – blood tests show digoxin levels below therapeutic level therefore digoxin increased to 0.375 mg daily. Enalapril 2.5 mg added twice daily to increase vasodilation. Fluid output equals intake.	31.7	Move bed nearer to toilet and encourage to walk. Sit out in chair for meals.
				31.7	Discontinue fluid balance chart.

Fig. 7.3 (continued)

Time and date	Problem		Progress and evaluation	Modification	
	P	Risk of falling	Has not fallen	31.7	Provide sticks for walking.
	P	Stiffness and immobility	No difficulty getting from bed to commode. Managing unaided.	31.7	Provide high chair for sitting.
	P	Increased joint pain	Remains pain free at rest and on present movement.		
	P	DVT	No signs of DVT.		
	P	Pressure sores	Skin intact. No pain or redness over pressure points.		

living, appears to concentrate largely on the physiological and physical aspects of the individual, though Roper *et al.* (1985) suggest that the psychological, cultural and social environment together with the age and level of dependence/independence can influence behaviour in the ALs. Annie's actual and potential problems appeared to be essentially physiological. She appeared to have adapted well to the constraints imposed on her life by breathlessness and osteoarthritis. She had a close relationship with her sister, enjoyed a comparatively active social life and rarely appeared anxious about her shortness of breath.

Although it is possible that a model such as Roy's (1984), by exploring self-concept, may have revealed more about her attitude to illness and disability we felt that the Roper model did allow for identification of Annie's problems. Assessing Annie's usual routines was particularly relevant and useful as it provided us with a yardstick by which to measure success. We felt it also stressed positive aspects of behaviour and revealed how well Annie was coping with disability. The problem-solving approach of the nursing process may be criticised for concentrating on negative aspects of patient behaviour, so consideration of positive aspects and coping mechanisms identified in assessment can be useful as a means of valuing what a person can already do and may make it possible to more accurately predict realistic dates for goal achievement.

The allowance in the model for the inclusion of potential problems such as deep vein thrombosis and pressure sores was important particularly in a work situation where untrained staff outnumber

trained staff and preventative measures need to be clearly incorporated into the care plans. Roper *et al.* (1981) recommend that problems, goals and nursing interventions are acceptable to the patient. This then should also lead to discussion about potential problems and the nursing interventions that might be appropriate. This can have the advantage, as it did with Annie, of a sense of involvement for the patient and a commitment to ensure goals are achieved. Furthermore in advocating assessment as an ongoing process (Roper *et al.*, 1981) potential problems should be anticipated.

Other users of Roper's model (Steward and Strachan, 1983) have reported some difficulty in deciding to which AL problems were related. Potential deep vein thrombosis and pressure sores for example may be related to the AL of maintaining a safe environment. However, as restricted mobility due to bed rest was felt to be the influencing factor these were included for Annie under the AL of mobility.

Identification of problems specifically linked to one or other AL, as described by Roper *et al.* (1985), was found to be a major constraint. Assessment highlighted a high level of interdependence between the ALs in terms of both actual and potential problems. Thus to separate problems in order to link them to particular ALs was felt to be artificial and insensitive to the wholeness of the individual. Similarly evaluation tended to focus on the whole person rather than on achievement of goals related to specific ALs. This was not the case however with the problem of breathlessness as this was a priority for Annie and thus stood out as important.

The planning stage of the nursing process according to Roper *et al.* (1985) involves the setting of goals and the selection of appropriate nursing actions to meet those goals. Goals should be written in observable or measureable terms. Some goals, such as those relating to the AL of breathing, had a short and long-term element incorporated as recommended by Kratz (1979). This allowed improvement to be measured at certain stages which were clearly identifiable to the patient and staff. Specific times by which goals were expected to be achieved were not always set as it was felt that a realistic time could not always be anticipated and the problem related to breathing, for example, was felt to depend partly on the patient's response to medication.

Roper *et al.* (1986) suggest planning care should be sensitive to available resources such as equipment, manpower and environment. This fits with the present climate which aims to match services to resources. Roper's model therefore may encourage nurses to use available resources imaginatively and may, for example, help to identify necessary skill mixes. For Annie's care planning it was essential to recognise that untrained staff would be involved in implementing the care plan. As stated earlier the identification of potential problems was seen as a particular strength of the model because it prepared the way for interventions to be clearly specified whose purpose was largely preventive. The choice of such interventions must remain the responsibility of qualified staff whose nursing knowledge should equip them to make informed decisions.

As the documentation demonstrates, the progress and evaluation record was used to document care given, and to evaluate goal achievement at the specified time and date. Roper *et al.* (1985) advocate the use of a progress sheet to record implementation and this was found to be useful in that it offered an ongoing summary of care given and changes occurring.

In conclusion it appeared that the use of the model was successful. All the problems were resolved though medical intervention with drugs played a part in reducing Annie's breathlessness. Roper, however, acknowledges the contribution to care made by medical intervention and recognises that some nursing actions will be linked to this. For example, measuring Annie's fluid intake and output and making recordings of her apex rate and respiratory rate provided a means of evaluating the effectiveness of the administration of frusemide and digoxin.

Annie expressed satisfaction with her involvement in the planning of care and maintained a clear commitment to the achievement of goals set. A willingness to include patients in the decision-making process about choices of nursing action probably reflects as much about nurses' attitudes to patient autonomy as it does about the nursing model used. However, using a model that values patient involvement should ensure that nurses give careful thought to the patient role. Roper's model can therefore be seen as one such.

Problem identification for Annie did emphasise the physical nature of the care required. Arguably Roper's model is most appropriate when problems are largely physical but there must remain concern that other problems may be missed or given less priority when organising care around a model that offers little scope for the assessment of psychological and social factors.

It was clear during the implementation of Roper's model that the concept of planning care around activities of living provided a similar emphasis to that derived from traditional ways of organising nursing care. In this particular instance, the care offered seemed to fit Annie's expectations of care in hospital. However, as Chavasse (1987) has identified, a growing number of people are demanding a more holistic approach to care and nurses will need to be sensitive to this demand when choosing a model of nursing.

References

Aggleton P & Chalmers H 1985 Roper's activities of living model. *Nursing Times*, February 13: 59–61.
Alderman C 1983 Individual care in action. *Nursing Times*, January 19: 15–17.
Chavasse JM 1987 A comparison of three models of nursing. *Nursing Education Today*, 7: 177–186.
Collins S & Parker E 1983 *An Introduction to Nursing.* Macmillan, London.
Cooke S 1982 Mr Jones has pump failure. *Nursing*, January: 1435–1439.

Du Gas B 1983 *Introduction to Patient Care.* WB Saunders Co, Philadelphia.

Durie M 1984 Respiratory problems and nursing intervention. *Nursing Series*, 2, 28: 826–828.

Herbert R 1984 Maintaining circulatory volume. *Nursing Series*, 2, 26: 76–78.

Henderson V 1966 *The Nature of Nursing.* Macmillan, New York.

Kershaw B & Salvage J (Eds) 1986 *Models for Nursing.* John Wiley & Sons, Chichester.

Kitchen I 1984 Congestive heart failure and cardiogenic shock: Drug therapy. *Nursing Series*, 2, 25: 243–245.

Kratz C 1979 *The Nursing Process.* Bailliere Tindall, London.

McGurn WC 1981 *People with cardiac problems: Nursing concepts.* Lippincott, Toronto.

Pearson A & Vaughan B 1986 *Nursing Models for Practice.* Heinemann, London.

Roper N, Logan W & Tierney A 1981 *Learning to Use the Process of Nursing.* Churchill Livingstone, Edinburgh.

Roper N, Logan W & Tierney A 1985 *The Elements of Nursing*, 2nd ed. Churchill Livingstone, Edinburgh.

Roper N, Logan W & Tierney A 1986 Nursing models: A process of construction and refinement. In *Models for Nursing,* B Kershaw & J Salvage (Eds). John Wiley & Sons, Chichester.

Roy C 1984 *Introduction to Nursing: Adaptation Model.* Prentice-Hall, Englewood Cliffs, New Jersey.

Stewart E & Strachan H 1983 A study in a surgical ward. In *Using a Model for Nursing,* N Roper, W Logan & A Tierney (Eds). Churchill Livingstone, Edinburgh.

Turner A & Turner J 1982 An unexpected killer. *Nursing Times*, August 25: 64–65.

Wilson-Barnett J 1986 From heart failure to independence. *Nursing Times*, January 22: 24–27.

8

Care plan for a man with chronic obstructive airways disease, using Roy's Adaptation model

Marie May

Introduction

This chapter presents the nursing care plan for a 76-year-old ex-miner suffering from chronic obstructive airways disease, and is based on Roy's Adaptation model (1980). Care takes place in a local community hospital.

Throughout the care plan only brief mention will be made of the acute stage of illness with which this man was admitted, attention being focused largely on the rehabilitation stage.

Review of the Literature

From a study of the literature available on the subject it seems that chronic obstructive airways disease is one of the commonest causes of absence from work in the United Kingdom. Sterling (1983) points out that it accounted for the loss of 30 million working days per annum in the mid-70s and the estimated figure for deaths per annum from the disease was 27,000.

The nomenclature of the disease includes chronic obstructive lung disease (COLD) and the term most widely used in American and Canadian literature, chronic obstructive pulmonary disease (COPD).

MacLeod (1984) describes chronic obstructive airways disease as a combination of chronic bronchitis and emphysema, characterised by a chronic cough and dyspnoea. Other experts also consider that asthma is a contributory factor. It has

been pointed out by Dalrymple (1984) that chronic obstructive airways disease can also be caused by other less common disorders such as bronchiectasis or cystic fibrosis.

Although the pathogenesis of chronic obstructive airways disease has not been clearly identified, there appears to be general agreement in current literature that cigarette smoking is a primary factor in its aetiology, together with other factors such as air pollution and the inhalation of dust particles.

It has been suggested by Crompton (1980) and Nett and Petty (1984) that there may also be an inherent predisposition for some people to develop chronic obstructive airways disease, including those who suffer from an alpha$_1$ antitrypsin deficiency state associated with chronic bronchitis and emphysema.

It is significant that current literature and clinical textbooks reveal a distinct change in attitude to nursing practice for patients with chronic obstructive airways disease. During acute exacerbations of chronic obstructive airways disease the individual's physiological and safety needs must not be neglected. This is emphasised by Duffy (1985). He sees the nurse's role at this stage as 'relieving breathlessness, preventing complications of respiratory failure and immobility, and promoting optimum comfort', and advocates that 'the nurses must work closely with the doctors in the initiation and management of the medical regime'. Nevertheless there is a move in nursing practice away from the medical model of nursing, which has a disease/treatment orientation, and towards a more holistic approach, where there is consideration of the psychological as well as the physiological factors influencing the patient's recovery. The ultimate aim is that of helping the patient with chronic obstructive airways disease to maintain a desired role within the family, home and society.

This 'desired' role is attained by increasing the patient's control over the symptoms, increasing exercise tolerance and improving self-esteem and feelings of worth. Nursing practice thus seems to be more rehabilitative, with the nurse's role being seen by many, including Burns (1983) as that of 'mentor and educator'.

One observation that is pertinent here is that many of these approaches to change in nursing practice, as well as research studies exploring the rehabilitative approach to patient care, are to be found mainly in literature from the USA and Canada. There appears to be little British nursing literature available on the rehabilitative approach to patient care in chronic obstructive airways disease, with the exception of textbooks written for physio-therapists.

Studies such as those conducted by Perry (1981) and Boyer *et al.* (1982) into the effectiveness of teaching in the rehabilitation of patients with chronic obstructive airways disease, indicated that a programme which included active patient involve-ment in self-care encouraged patients to make decisions and increased their ability to cope with their illness. However, Perry (1981) acknowledges that further research is necessary to ascertain the effects over a longer period of time, and Boyer *et al.* (1982) note that where there is increased severity of illness there is a parallel decrease in patient success. Nevertheless, in most of the literature studied, breathing retraining, such as abdominal breathing, pursed-lips exhalation, and prolonged exhalation, seems to be one of the major areas where nurses, in conjunction with physiotherapists, are seen to play the role of teacher.

The importance of the nurse's role in respiratory rehabilitation is stressed by Burns (1983), who sees the nurse as a catalyst in the process of maximising physiological and psychological improvement and increasing the patient's level of motivation. This appears to be of critical importance in reducing the emotional trauma of anger, frustration, regression

and apathy, and therefore, according to Mascher (1984), 'enables the patient to maintain a reason-able degree of self-worth and autonomy'.

Nursing practice also includes the role of health educator, for example, in the area of nutrition. Correcting nutritional deficits is seen by Curgian and Pagano (1985) as paramount in the manage-ment of chronic obstructive airways disease. They point out that apart from the extra calories needed to compensate for extra energy used in the effort of breathing, there is 'direct correlation between malnutrition and an increased susceptibility to infection' (Curgian and Pagano, 1985). Burns (1983), Dalrymple (1984) and De Vito (1985), among others, also support the value of adequate nutrition and the need for the nurse to help the patient to achieve this goal by appropriate teaching.

Other agreed health measures about which the nurse can help to increase understanding are infection control, sleep and rest. Sleep and rest are seen as particularly important, since damaged lungs need extra energy to meet the body's demand for oxygen. Sjoberg (1983) says that 'sleep is essential for clients with lung disease'. Although sleep disturbance in patients with chronic obstructive airways disease may be caused by several factors, including breathing difficulties, treatment regime, anxiety and environment, throughout the literature the nurse is encouraged to play a major role in diagnosing the cause of sleep disturbance and taking appropriate action.

The literature recommends liaison between the patient, his or her family and the nurse to help the patient and family adjust to changes in their roles and their lives in general. Thus skills of com-munication and forming relationships are essential if nurses are to be effective.

To sum up, the nurse's role is that of encourag-ing rehabilitation, particularly helping the patient to overcome ineffective patterns of breathing. It appears that when patients with chronic obstructive airways disease are finding breathing easier some of their related social and emotional problems dis-appear, and those social and emotional problems which remain may then be focused upon more effectively by the nurse.

Justification for choice of model

The consensus of opinion among the contributors to the literature studied on the subject of nursing care for those with a medical diagnosis of chronic obstructive airways disease is that nurses should be encouraged to look beyond the immediate physiological needs of the patient and explore how insights from understanding psychological and social needs may aid the planning and delivery of care. It was therefore decided that Roy's Adaptation model (1980) would be the most appropriate model to use in undertaking the care of Mr N.

The use of Roy's model also fitted well with the notion put forward by Sexton (1981) that 'chronic illness precipitates a process of adaptation', as Roy's model uses an approach that focuses on individuals who are having difficulty coping with changes in their lives.

A further recommendation is that this model also uses a problem-solving approach to assist and support people in achieving adaptive states, which links well with the trend towards rehabilitation and learning, with the nurse acting as mentor and educator.

The focus on self-concept, role function and interdependence which characterises the Roy model also seemed particularly suitable for this patient, as the changes in life-style and body image caused by the progressive nature of chronic obstructive airways disease can lead to a loss of self-esteem and worth.

The model was also chosen because it acknowledges the importance of past events and experiences on the present situation. According to Roy (1980) such residual stimuli will influence current behaviour. It was felt that for Mr N previous exacerbations of chronic obstructive airways disease, earlier hospital admissions and his wife's death could all influence his behaviour and this in turn would affect the planning and delivery of nursing care.

Description and critique of chosen model

Roberts and Roy (1981) describe the recipient of nursing care as an adaptive system, and Tiedeman (1983) sees the central components of Roy's model as the concepts of person, adaptation, nursing, health–illness and environment.

Roy (1980) views her model primarily as a systems model with an interactionist level of analysis. The person is thought of as having parts or elements linked together in such a way that force on the linkages can be increased or decreased. Increased force or tension comes from strains within the system or the environment which impinge on that system. These changes, which demand a response, are stressors or focal stimuli, and are mediated by contextual or residual factors. Roy describes focal stimuli as those immediately confronting the individual, contextual stimuli as all the other stimuli present and residual stimuli as being those from past learning and its effects. Such residual stimuli then become beliefs and values.

Roy further describes the individual as a bio-psychosocial being who strives for homeostasis by attempting to balance the constant interaction between the internal and external environments. However, although environment seems to be fairly well defined the distinction between internal and external environment is not clear. Roberts and Roy (1981) acknowledge this by saying that 'further clarification of environment as distinct from internal stimuli awaits additional theoretical work on the model'.

Roy (1980) suggests that the system of the person and his or her interaction with the environment are the units of analysis of nursing assessment, and that nursing intervention should consist of manipulation either of parts of the environment or parts of the system or person. This has now been revised by Roberts and Roy (1981) to indicate that intervention should consist of manipulation of stimuli which they argue is different from manipulating people. No clear example has been given of this, and it is difficult to see how residual stimuli can be manipulated without manipulating the person.

The adaptation concept central to this model follows the work of Helson (1964) which saw a person's ability to adapt as dependent both upon the stimulus and the individual's adaptation level resulting from the pooled effects of focal, contextual and residual stimuli. Roy describes this positive adaptation level as a zone indicating the range of stimulation that will lead to a positive response. However, Fawcett (1984) suggests that the major premise, namely that the person is an adaptive system, is yet to be empirically supported.

Roberts and Roy (1981) explain that regulation of the focal stimuli (by increasing, decreasing or maintaining stimulation) may cause them to fall within the adaptation level, while manipulation of contextual and residual stimuli may broaden the adaptive zone.

According to Roy's model, positive adaptations are those responses which promote integrity and health in terms of the goals of survival, growth, reproduction and mastery. Negative adaptation would result in behaviour that would not contribute to these goals.

Roy believes that to cope with or adapt to stress created by a changing environment, individuals use both innate and acquired mechanisms which are biological, social and psychological in origin. These mechanisms consist of both regulator or autonomic nervous system activity, and cognator activity which consists of conscious decision-making, or unconscious defence mechanism action. Although Roy (1984) describes the action of cognator and regulator coping mechanisms she recognises that much work is still needed to gain a greater understanding of these processes.

Secondary to this cognator and regulator activity, Roberts and Roy (1981) describe four modes of adaptation: physiological, self-concept, interdependence and role function. The physiological mode allows the nurse to view the client from the more medically orientated perspective supported by some nursing models, while the other three modes would seem to incorporate an interactionist view.

The Roy model allows for recognition of a person both as an individual and as part of a family and community, and sees these as inseparable. The inseparability of past from present is also acknowledged with recognition of the influence of residual stimuli on present behaviour. For instance, Burns and Kinney (1983), in using Roy's model when caring for a patient with asthma, found one residual stimulus which may have been affecting the patient's behaviour was the possible relationship between unresolved grief and the initial onset of asthma 16 years before.

It is claimed by Roberts and Roy (1981) that the Roy model has been 'more fully developed and operationalised' than some other models. Among early work illustrating how Roy's model could be applied was that of Starr (1980), who used the model when caring for a dying patient, and Schmitz (1980), who showed how Roy's model could be applied in a community setting. Rambo (1984), found it to be a workable and useful model in a variety of settings with considerable potential for flexibility in meeting patients' needs.

More recently the flexibility of Roy's model has been demonstrated by Dobratz (1984) in caring for a dying patient or 'Life Closure'. The assumption that health and illness are an inevitable part of a person's life was broadened to include death, thus restating the assumption to suggest 'that each person is subject to the laws of health, illness and death'. Dobratz (1984) also incorporated within her broadened continuum a closure continuum in which defined stages of behaviour identified by Kubler-Ross (1970) could be placed when assessed behaviours were recognised.

However, this seems a rather complicated interpretation of Roy's model. Although Dobratz (1984) and Kubler-Ross (1970) suggest that behaviours exhibited by patients will not follow a set pattern, Dobratz defines closure continuum as 'a continuum that shows a progression through defined and accepted stages of behaviour from impending death to finality of life'.

Such an approach has a somewhat rigid and mechanistic flavour. On the other hand, Chadderton's (1986) use of Roy's model in caring for someone who is terminally ill was clearer and reflected more sensitively the concerns of Roy's (1980) model. In common with other works mentioned here, however, it is not clear who defines the person's position on the health–illness continuum. Does the definition of extreme poor health depend on the nurse's perception or the patient's opinion? Such a decision is of course crucial to the planning of patient care. Given the commitment to an interactionist approach (Roy, 1980), nurses may need to explore the value of negotiation when trying to establish an individual's position on the health–illness continuum.

In Roy's model there is no clear definition of what constitutes wellness, though Fawcett (1984) points out that Roy mentions maximum, peak and high-level wellness. In addition, there is no explicit definition of illness, so that it must be inferred that an adaptive response means wellness and an ineffective response suggests illness. Tiedeman (1983) believes that the concepts of health and illness within Roy's model need more attention and further clarification. Fawcett (1984) further criticises Roy in that she suggests that the classification of the person's responses as adaptive or ineffective implies a dichotomy rather than a continuum. Hammond and Mastal (1980) have tried to modify in some measure the health–illness continuum by adding stages of transition which link to societal norms for health and illness behaviours. It is not, however, within Roy's model alone that problems exist when trying to measure health and illness or when trying to identify and evaluate the usefulness of supposed societal norms.

Evaluation of use of model

The model will be evaluated by looking at Mr N's care within the context of the nursing process and the Roy Adaptation model.

The Roy Adaptation model includes a detailed nursing process and Roy (1984) identifies six steps in the application of the nursing process, namely the first and second level assessments, nursing diagnosis, goal-setting, intervention and evaluation. This framework was used to implement care for Mr N, and the format of the care plan is similar to that presented by Schmitz (1980). Some of the care plan is written in patient terms, which would be in keeping with Roy's own view of the patient being actively involved.

According to Roy (1984), in the first level assessment the nurse systematically looks at behaviour in each adaptive mode. However, in practice, when admitting Mr N the behaviours in all the modes could not be adequately assessed as Mr N was too breathless and frightened to communicate verbally and his non-verbal communication was concentrated on demonstrating his distress. Thus the first level assessment which Roy (1980) says may be carried out rapidly was in fact completed over a period of 24 hours (Fig. 8.1). This did not prevent nursing staff from using observational skills to note, for example, dehydration and weight-loss in the physiological mode. The patient's perception of why these maladaptive behaviours had occurred was ascertained later.

Some of the behaviours identified seemed to relate to more than one mode, a difficulty which Roy acknowledges. One example of this was the feeling of uselessness identified in the self-concept mode, which was also seen as ineffective behaviour in the role function mode. Another difficulty concerned Mr N's loneliness. Worden (1983) sees loneliness following bereavement as normal, which would suggest it to be an adaptive behaviour. However, discussion identified that Mr N perceived loneliness to be a problem and so it was considered in the interdependence mode although both Mr N and the nurse acknowledged that it could affect behaviour in other modes as well.

Two particular adaptive behaviours were considered in the physiological mode, as Roy (1984) suggests that the nurse should also be interested in adaptive as well as ineffective behaviour. In this instance it was felt that these adaptive behaviours would be a guideline for the nurse helping Mr N to cope with the changes brought about by his present illness, and thus encourage adaptation.

Despite problems encountered in deciding which ineffective behaviour should be associated with which mode, the first level assessment yielded some useful data. Roy (1984) acknowledges the preliminary nature of the first level assessment and allows that at its completion it may only be possible to make tentative judgements about whether behaviour is adaptive or not.

The contribution of the second level assessment is therefore particularly important. It offers an invaluable opportunity to enhance the nurse–patient relationship and encourages both validation with the patient of behaviours noted during the first

Fig. 8.1 First level behavioural assessment

PHYSIOLOGICAL MODE	
Exercise and rest	Feels tired. Mr N usually manages gardening and shopping. Exercise curtailed over last month due to breathlessness. Cannot get to sleep as he is worried about breathless attacks during the night. Has woken twice nightly for last month with breathlessness.
Nutrition	Poor appetite. He feels he cannot get his breath long enough to eat. This has got worse over the last month. Says he has lost weight.
Elimination	Says he is constipated. Usually has bowels open daily. Has missed 4 days now. Urine volume seems unchanged to Mr N.
Fluids and electrolytes	Feels too breathless to drink. Skin dry and lacks elasticity.
Oxygen and circulation	Respirations 38 per minute. Has cough and audible wheeze. Is producing unpleasant sputum. Distressed by breathlessness. Says inhaler not helping. Pulse 120 per minute. BP 190/90.
Endocrine and sensory regulation	Temperature 37°C. Senses: vision poor, hearing normal. Senses of taste, touch and smell not tested. Endocrine system: no apparent problems.
SELF-CONCEPT MODE	
Physical self	Is unable to do things for himself at present. Feels 'useless'. Very weepy about this. Concerned about loss of weight over last 8 months.
Personal self	Anxious about increased breathlessness. Looks unhappy. Dislikes nurses doing things for him, particularly assisting him to hold urinal while he passes water.
Interpersonal self	Finding it difficult to communicate verbally because talking makes him breathless.
ROLE FUNCTION MODE	A widower. Feels he 'won't be the same after this setback'. Wants to be able to look after his garden which he loves. Does not know how he is going to cope.
INTERDEPENDENCE MODE	Lives alone. 'I am lonely since my wife died 14 months ago. I still miss her.'

stage and an increase in the amount of data available on which to base decisions.

Roy (1984) sees the second level assessment centred on a search for factors (stimuli) influencing, or possibly causing, the maladaptive behaviour. Again, this assessment had to be carried out in stages for Mr N (Fig. 8.2). This is not out of keeping with Roy's method, which recognises that situational variables may mean that certain behaviours are considered first. So focal, contextual and residual stimuli affecting oxygen and circulation needs in the physiological mode were identified first because these were thought to threaten Mr N's physiological safety. Some difficulty was encountered in identifying contextual and residual stimuli, but Roy (1984) suggests that these particular distinctions are less important than the nurse coming to a greater understanding of the patient as a whole.

According to Roy (1984) a nursing diagnosis is the nurse's interpretation of the assessment data and may include prioritising the problems identified. Although not explicitly advocated by Roy, Mr N's participation in this prioritisation and the subsequent selection of nursing actions was encouraged.

Fig. 8.2 Second level behavioural assessment

Mode	Focal stimuli	Contextual stimuli	Residual stimuli
PHYSIOLOGICAL			
Exercise and rest			
Mr N feels very tired.	Lack of sleep.	Woken by breathlessness. Anxious about being breathless at night. Is alone at night.	Believes he will get breathless each night. Wife died during the night in this hospital.
Reduced ability to take exercise.	Breathless on exertion.	Chronic obstructive airways disease. Observed using inhaler incorrectly.	Believes nothing can help the breathlessness.
Nutrition			
Poor appetite. Weight loss.	Too breathless to eat.	Chronic obstructive airways disease. Unpleasant sputum leaves nasty taste in mouth.	Not very interested in preparing food since wife's death. Associates eating with becoming breathless.
Elimination			
Constipated.	Finds it difficult to get to lavatory.	Breathlessness. Poor diet. Low fluid intake.	Apparently unaware of major influence of diet on bowel action.
Fluids and electrolytes			
Not drinking adequate amounts.	Breathless when drinking.	Chronic obstructive airways disease.	
Oxygen and circulation			
Breathless. Coughing up unpleasant sputum.	Exacerbation of chronic obstructive airways disease. Chest infection.	Coal miner for 40 years.	Believes he might die. Both wife and son died in this hospital.

The goal of nursing intervention put forward by Roy (1984) is to maintain and enhance adaptive behaviours, and to change ineffective behaviours to adaptive ones. She advocates that goals should be realistic, whether short-term or long-term. All goals set were patient-centred as this offers a significant means of achieving patient involvement in care and deliberately focuses evaluation on changes in patient behaviour. In practice the setting of patient-centred goals was found to be most effective in gaining Mr N's confidence as he could readily anticipate the progress he might make. This was especially useful once Mr N began to be more mobile and was regarded, and regarded himself, as rehabilitating.

Goal setting in the role function mode was delayed because discussing his future clearly distressed Mr N during the period when problems in the physiological mode were paramount. The idea that the meeting of basic survival needs must take place before other needs can be usefully addressed is supported by Maslow (1954) among

Fig. 8.2 (continued)

Mode	Focal stimuli	Contextual stimuli	Residual stimuli
SELF-CONCEPT			
Physical self			
Feels useless and this upsets him.	Does not feel well enough to look after himself.	Now in hospital. Nurses are doing things for him.	Believes physical dependence means he is useless.
Worried about his increasing weight loss.	Recent weight loss.	Poor appetite. Breathlessness. Has to cook his own meals.	Sees weight loss as a sign of poor health.
Personal self			
Anxious about his increasing breathlessness.	Increasing breathlessness.		Believes he has got worse since his wife died.
Seems depressed.		Current poor health. Bereavement.	(Depression may be adaptive as part of the grieving process but may accompany anxiety (Burns and Kinney, 1983).)
Dislikes nurses doing things for him.	Particularly dislikes having help when passing water.		Has expectations of self that preclude help with certain personal functions. Likes privacy.
Interpersonal self			
Difficulty in talking very much at a time.	Breathlessness.	Hospital. Aware of other ill patients.	Believes nurses are too busy to spend a lot of time with him.
ROLE FUNCTION			
Worried at how he is going to manage his home and garden.	Feels powerless.	Nurses are helping him a lot.	
INTERDEPENDENCE			
Lonely	Death of wife.	Lives alone. Sees wives visiting other patients.	His wife was his main companion.

others. Furthermore, goals were not set in the interdependence mode as Mr N was unwilling to talk about his wife. This may have been due to inexperience on the part of staff in coping with a bereaved person, but when more adaptive behaviours were reached in other modes Mr N did discuss his wife more frequently and apparently with greater ease.

In the intervention stage of the nursing process the nurse acts to manage the stimuli affecting behaviour. Roy (1984) suggests that this involves broadening the adaptation level by changing the other stimuli present. The initial intervention to promote adaptation was that of relieving Mr N's dyspnoea. Adaptive behaviour was obtained, and intervention leading to more effective behaviours in other modes could then proceed.

Roy (1984) sees the final step of the nursing process as the evaluation of the effectiveness of nursing intervention. This effectiveness is judged by reconsidering the behaviour demonstrated in each adaptive mode.

Evaluation of goals set with Mr N took place in all modes and most goals had been met (Fig. 8.3). However, Mr N did not gain weight. He appeared to be eating better by the time he was discharged and in retrospect a goal to maintain his present weight might have been more realistic.

Roy's model proved a very useful and flexible model in caring for Mr N. The two-level assessment offered an opportunity to explore possible reasons for ineffective behaviours and at the same time to establish empathy with Mr N, which was valuable in his subsequent care. The assessment in

Fig. 8.3 Care plan

Nursing diagnosis	Goal	Intervention	Evaluation/modification
Breathlessness	Mr N will breathe more easily as soon as possible, demonstrated by lowered respiratory rate.	Administer GP prescribed drugs and oxygen. Sit Mr N well up in bed. Nurse to remain with Mr N to observe and encourage him.	*At 1 hour* Respiratory rate 30 per minute. Continue planned interventions.
Using inhaler incorrectly.	Within 3 days Mr N will correctly demonstrate use of inhaler.	Nurse to explain and demonstrate inhaler use once Mr N is feeling less breathless. Nurse to observe Mr N using inhaler and give feedback on performance.	Mr N showing adaptive behaviour and using inhaler correctly. Mr N pleased that inhaler seems more effective.
Constipation	Mr N will have his bowels open during next 4 hours.	Nurse will administer enema if rectal examination shows full rectum. (Gastrointestinal distension can elevate diaphragm and restrict breathing. (Dalrymple, 1984).)	Bowels open. Further adaptive behaviour required to improve fibre and fluid intake. (Use of enemas is seen as maladaptive by Rambo (1984).)
	Mr N will eat sufficient high-fibre food and will have a fluid intake of 1500 ml/24 hours in order to re-establish a regular bowel action (1 week).	Nursing staff to assist Mr N in his menu choice and to provide sufficient fluids that he likes.	Mr N now having his bowels open with minimal effort on alternate days.
Weight loss	Mr N will gain 3 lb per week for 3 weeks.	Nurse to encourage Mr N to eat a nutritious diet. Also to encourage small frequent meals once acute breathlessness is improved.	*1 week* Mr N continues to show maladaptive behaviour – refuses food. No weight gain. *Reassess* Consider whether poor eating is a sign of grief (Parkes, 1975).
Feeling useless	By 1 week Mr N will state he feels of some use.	Nurse and physiotherapist to help Mr N regain exercise tolerance by (i) teaching techniques that maximise breathing capacity (Mascher, 1984); (ii) planning with Mr N a programme of increasing activity.	Mr N says he can now wash himself and so he feels useful. Continue intervention as planned.

Fig. 8.3 (continued)

Nursing diagnosis	Goal	Intervention	Evaluation/modification
	By discharge Mr N will feel better about himself and will make positive statements about the physical things he can do.		*On discharge* Demonstrating adaptive behaviour. Walking about the ward and hospital without getting too breathless. Talking cheerfully to staff and patients. Says he is able to do many of the things that now matter to him.
Feels tired	Mr N will state he feels less tired by 1 week.	Breathlessness to be controlled as above. Nurses to encourage Mr N to establish which position is most comfortable in bed (Gaskell and Webber, 1980).	Mr N still feels tired. Continue interventions as planned.
	By discharge Mr N will achieve a sleep pattern that he is happy with. (Sjoberg (1983) identifies sleep as critical when lungs are damaged.)	Nurses to reduce environmental stimuli that Mr N finds obtrusive. Physiotherapist to teach controlled breathing to reduce anxiety. In the event of breathlessness a nurse to remain with Mr N to allay anxiety.	*On discharge* Some night-time breathlessness still occurring. Episodes decreasing in frequency. Mr N says he is less tired and feels he is sleeping well enough. Thinks he will cope with occasional night-time breathlessness at home.
Worried about how he is going to manage his home and garden	Mr N will adapt to changing ability to manage by indicating other ways of coping.	Nurse to offer the opportunity to discuss what has to be done at Mr N's home and in his garden. Nurse to encourage Mr N to explore alternative strategies for managing his home and garden and to discuss ways in which he can maximise his own potential. Social worker to join discussions if possible.	Mr N showing enthusiasm for actively managing the care of his home and garden even if he does not do all the physical work himself. Has refused meals-on-wheels but will consider home help. Mr N has met social worker once for discussions about help available.

four modes provided a comprehensive basis for investigation of the patient's situation in a more holistic way than seems possible with the medical model or nursing models with a heavy biological emphasis. Thus, although Mr N was admitted for physiological reasons, nursing investigation revealed important adaptation problems in other modes.

It was expected that the identification of residual stimuli would highlight the significance of the past experiences brought to any situation by an individual. In the event two major lessons were learned. Firstly, the identification of residual stimuli is difficult and the extent of their impact on a given situation is similarly problematic. When caring for Mr N certain assumptions were made about the relevance of the deaths of both his wife and son in the same hospital, and the effect this might have on his present attitudes to care. There is certainly nursing literature (Jasmin and Trygstad, 1979) to support the notion that past experiences influence attitudes but the relationship in Mr N's case was never satisfactorily clarified.

Secondly, the past experiences of the nursing staff were also important. As has been mentioned above, a lack of experience in talking to bereaved people may have influenced the quality of the data collected from Mr N in the interdependence mode.

The choice of nursing model is not value-free. Roy (1980) advocates nursing interventions that manipulate stimuli. If residual stimuli are thought of as beliefs, attitudes and values, then nurses may find themselves attempting to change these. This may raise ethical questions. Richardson (1977), for example, holds the view that what one believes usually provides a most accurate and reliable basis for action. Nurses working with Roy's model will need to consider carefully the implications of working with a model with such a possible emphasis during intervention.

References

Boyer M, Brough FK, Rasmussen T & Schmidt CD 1982 Comparison of two teaching methods for self-care training for patients with chronic obstructive pulmonary disease. *Patient Counselling and Health Education*, 4, 2: 111–115.

Burns MD 1983 *Pulmonary Care: A Guide to Patient Education.* Appleton-Century-Crofts, Norwalk.

Burns MD & Kinney N 1983 Use of the Roy adaptation model in the study of a patient with asthma. In *Pulmonary care: a guide to patient education*, MD Burns. Appleton-Century-Crofts, Norwalk.

Chadderton H 1986 A stress adaptation model in terminal care. In *Models for Nursing*, B Kershaw & J Salvage (Eds). John Wiley & Sons, Chichester.

Crompton GK 1980 *Diagnosis and Management of Respiratory Diseases.* Blackwell Scientific Publications, Oxford.

Curgian LM & Pagano K 1985 Nutrition in chronic respiratory disease. *Rehabilitation Nursing*, 10, 6: 22–23.

Dalrymple DL 1984 Compensating for COPD. In *Respiratory Disorders*, T Ford et al. (Eds). Springhouse Corporation, Pennsylvania.

De Vito A 1985 Rehabilitation of patients with chronic obstructive pulmonary disease. *Rehabilitation Nursing*, 10, 2: 12–15.

Dobratz MC 1984 Life closure. In *Introduction to Nursing: An Adaptation Model*, C Roy (Ed). Prentice-Hall, Englewood Cliffs, New Jersey.

Duffy B 1985 Chronic breathing difficulties. *Nursing Mirror*, 161, 13: 40–42.

Fawcett J 1984 *Analysis and Evaluation of Conceptual Models of Nursing.* FA Davis, Philadelphia.

Gaskell DV & Webber BA 1980 *The Brompton Hospital Guide to Chest Physiotherapy.* Blackwell Scientific Publications, Oxford.

Hammond H & Mastal MF 1980 Analysis and expansion of the Roy adaptation model: a contribution to holistic nursing. *Advances in Nursing Science*, 2, 4: 71–81.

Helson H 1964 *Adaptation Level Theory: An Experimental and Systematic Approach to Behaviour.* Harper & Row, New York.

Jasmin S & Trygstad LN 1979 *Behavioural Concepts and the Nursing Process.* CV Mosby, London.

Kubler-Ross E 1970 *On Death and Dying.* Tavistock, London.

Macleod J (Ed) 1984 *Davidson's Principles and Practice of Medicine.* Churchill Livingstone, Edinburgh.

Mascher LD 1984 Helping exercises for your COPD patient. *Registered Nursing*, 47, 6: 33–35.

Maslow AH 1954 *Motivation and Personality.* Harper & Row, New York.

Nett LM & Petty TL 1984 *Enjoying Life with Emphysema.* Lea & Felinger, Philadelphia.

Parkes CM 1975 *Bereavement.* Penguin, Harmondsworth.

Perry JA 1981 Effectiveness of teaching in rehabilitation of patients with chronic bronchitis and emphysema. *Nursing Research*, 30, 4: 219–228.

Rambo B 1984 *Adaptation Nursing: Assessment and Intervention.* WB Saunders, Philadelphia.

Richardson A 1977 Attitudes. In *Introductory Psychology*, JC Coleman (Ed). Routledge & Kegan Paul, London.

Roberts SL & Roy C 1981 *Theory Construction in Nursing: An Adaptation Model.* Prentice-Hall, Englewood Cliffs, New Jersey.

Roy C 1980 The Roy adaptation model. In *Conceptual Models for Nursing Practice*, JP Riehl & C Roy (Eds). Appleton-Century-Crofts, Norwalk.

Roy C (ed) 1984 *Introduction to Nursing: An Adaptation Model*, Prentice-Hall, Englewood Cliffs, New Jersey.

Roy C 1984 The Roy model nursing process. In *Introduction to Nursing: An Adaptation Model*, C Roy (Ed). Prentice-Hall, Englewood Cliffs, New Jersey.

Schmitz M 1980 The Roy adaptation model: application in a community setting. In *Conceptual Models for Nursing Practice*, JP Riehl & C Roy (Eds). Appleton-Century-Crofts, Norwalk.

Sexton DL 1981 *Chronic Obstructive Pulmonary Disease: Care of the Child and Adult.* CV Mosby, St Louis.

Sjoberg EL 1983 Nursing diagnosis and the COPD patient. *American Journal of Nursing*, 83, 2: 244–248.

Starr SL 1980 Adaptation applied to the dying client. In *Conceptual Models for Nursing Practice*, JP Riehl & C Roy (Eds). Appleton-Century-Crofts, Norwalk.

Sterling GM 1983 *Respiratory disease.* Heinemann Medical, London.

Tiedeman ME 1983 The Roy adaptation model. In *Conceptual Models for Nursing: Analysis and Application*, JJ Fitzpatrick & AL Whall (Eds). Robert J Brady Co, Maryland.

Worden J 1983 *Grief Counselling and Grief Therapy.* Tavistock, London.

9

Care plan for a toddler with croup, using Henderson's Fundamental Needs model

Margaret Doman

Introduction

This chapter considers the nursing care given to 14-month-old Jamie T who was admitted to a paediatric ward on a July evening with croup. He was accompanied by his mother. Care is based on Henderson's model of nursing in preference to others due to her emphasis on the nurse's role in maintaining or restoring an individual's independence in meeting fundamental needs. For a child, these needs are usually met by the mother and father, according to Sacharin (1980). When caring for sick children, therefore, the parent(s) and child should be considered as an independent unit, with nursing intervention aiming to restore independence to the family unit (Watson, 1983). This was the overall goal in planning care for Jamie and his mother.

Since difficulty in breathing was the greatest problem for Jamie, the main aim of nursing action was to help him breathe more easily and ultimately for him to breathe normally again. This involved helping to calm both Jamie and his mother as soon as they arrived, and observing him closely (Barrell and Barnes, 1985) in order to detect any changes which could lead to a need for further action or for medical involvement.

The importance of parental involvement in the care of children in hospital was first recognised by the Department of Health and Social Security (DHSS) in the Platt Report in 1959 following work by Bowlby (1951) on maternal deprivation and the possible long-term psychological effects of hospital admission on a child. Burr (1984) suggests that since then, paediatric nurses have welcomed the concept of 'family-orientated care' and facilities have been made available for parents to stay with their sick children in most areas. For a child with croup, King and David (1982) and Coles (1977) firmly advocate the presence of a parent, for the child will breathe better if he is happy or asleep. It was therefore important for us to help alleviate Jamie's fears of hospital admission or separation from his mother, since, as Waechter and Blake (1976) point out, a child who is frightened or crying may exacerbate laryngospasm, producing a vicious circle.

Careful observation is the nurse's main role, state Barrell and Barnes (1985), and this should include frequent recording of pulse and respirations, and observing for increasing restlessness, intercostal and subcostal recession and pallor or cyanosis. Such observations can be carried out without disturbing the child. King and David (1982) stress the importance of reporting the presence of any of these symptoms when they accompany increasing pulse and respiratory rates, as this may indicate exhaustion and hypoxia which could result in respiratory arrest. Indeed they add that croup can be fatal if deterioration is not recognised. Cold mist is advocated by Coles (1977), possibly with an increased oxygen supply and the child being nursed in a tent and carefully observed. Milner (1984) believes, however, that cold mist is of no benefit since it distresses the child and has little effect on humidity in the larynx. He continues that ultrasonically-produced mist may actually increase airway obstruction in some children. Waechter and Blake (1976) add that cold moisture can create a cold, clammy atmosphere which is very unpleasant for the child, and croupettes can mist up and hide a child from view.

In the unit where Jamie was nursed, croupettes are provided and may be used for children admitted with croup. However, the noise generated by the air compressor, the physical separation from the mother and the clear plastic tents into which children are placed can increase distress (Barrell and Barnes, 1985) and may exacerbate breathing difficulties. Jamie was therefore helped to settle to sleep in his mother's arms, close to the croupette, and Mrs T herself decided to place him within the tent, keeping her own head and shoulders inside with him in case he should awake. Later in the night she took him into bed with her, where they both managed to get some sleep.

Close cooperation between nurses, doctors and other health carers is vital in paediatric nursing if the special needs of the whole child are to be met (Jolly, 1981). As yet no model exists specifically for the care of children, and Miles (1985) suggests that children's nursing still relies heavily on the medical model. This is a rather pessimistic view considering the advances made by paediatric nurses in implementing individualised care and family involvement (Burr, 1984), and the successful use of the models of Roy (1980) and Orem (1980) in caring for children (e.g., Evans, 1985; Eichelberger *et al.*, 1980).

Adam (1980) states that Henderson sees nursing as an independent health profession, but she also advocates a team approach in delivering care in which all carers (such as nurses, doctors, family, social workers, teachers, nursery nurses or physiotherapists) have a greater or lesser part to play (Henderson, 1972).

Individualised care is essential in paediatric nursing (Watson, 1983), since the needs of every child are very different, no matter what the reason for their admission to hospital. Patient allocation therefore exists throughout this paediatric unit, with mothers (and/or fathers) being encouraged to stay and help care for their children, thus helping to prevent psychological stress to the child. Henderson (1966) stresses the importance of nursing care recognising a person's individual needs, and acknowledging the autonomy of the patient (or, for children, the family unit) in planning and delivery of care. In addition, Chinn and Jacobs (1983) state that Henderson believes there is always a role for the family in health care, although she does not offer clear guidelines about the way this should be carried out.

Henderson's (1966) model of nursing emphasises the nurse's role in maintaining or restoring an individual's (or family unit's) independence in meeting fundamental needs. This aspect, considered alongside her acceptance of family involvement and patient autonomy, led to this model being chosen as a basis for the planning and delivery of Jamie's (and his mother's) care whilst in hospital.

Description of the model

In constructing her model of nursing, Henderson (1966) based some of her views of people on work by psychologists such as Thorndike (1940) and Maslow (1954) who see individuals as integrated wholes. Henderson (1964) also developed an analytical approach to all aspects of care and treatment, leading to an appreciation of the importance of physiological balance. In addition, she gained much experience in rehabilitation where many of her ideas of individualised programmes of care progressing ultimately towards independence were implemented.

Henderson's (1966) model is a systems model and Adam (1980) states that Henderson believes all individuals strive for, and desire, independence. She continues that all individuals are complex wholes with fourteen fundamental needs common to all human beings, be they sick or well. Those needs are to:

1 breathe normally;
2 eat and drink adequately;
3 eliminate body waste;
4 move and maintain desirable postures;
5 sleep and rest;
6 select suitable clothes – dress and undress;
7 maintain body temperature within normal range;

8   keep the body clean and well groomed;

9   avoid dangers in the environment, avoid injuring others;

10   communicate with others;

11   worship according to one's faith;

12   work in such a way that there is a sense of accomplishment;

13   play or participate in forms of recreation;

14   learn, discover and satisfy curiosity.

Fitzpatrick and Whall (1983) point out that Henderson believes health to be an individual's ability to be independent in attaining these fundamental needs, and that when a need is not satisfied, the person is no longer complete, whole or independent. Adam (1980) explains that to Henderson a 'need' is a requirement rather than a lack, and suggests that each need has biophysiological and psychosociocultural dimensions. Thus, despite these fundamental needs being common to all, individuals are unique in the way they meet or express them. Buchanan (1983) points out that this is especially true for children, who are individuals at a period of life during which major physical, psychological, social and educational developments take place even if the child is ill.

Henderson (1972) sees nursing as an independent health profession forming part of the health team, its 'unique function' being to

assist the individual, sick or well, in the performance of those activities contributing to health (or to peaceful death) that he would perform unaided if he had the necessary strength, will or knowledge.

In outlining the nursing activities involved, Henderson (1966) identifies fourteen components of basic nursing which relate to each of the fourteen fundamental needs. The aim of nursing care, according to Henderson, is to maintain or restore an individual's independence in satisfying these needs as rapidly as possible, thus clarifying the nurse's specific contribution to the preservation and improvement of health.

As already stated, for a child, fundamental needs are usually met by parents (Sacharin, 1980), so nursing intervention is not normally needed. When caring for sick children, therefore, Watson (1983)

suggests an overall goal of re-establishing the independence of the family unit.

Henderson does not specifically advocate use of the nursing process, but she considers (1972) that assessment of the patient's needs should involve negotiation between patient (or in this case, the family unit) and nurse in order to decide what needs are not being satisfied and whether assistance is necessary.

For Jamie, a nursing assessment was obtained from him and Mrs T by working through each fundamental need to establish Jamie's normal routine and identify where any problems or unsatisfied needs existed (Fig. 9.1). Brunner and Suddarth (1986) point out that when parents are active participants in their child's care they too have certain needs, so Mrs T's particular communication and learning needs were also documented.

Adam (1980) states that Henderson believes a nurse is committed to solving or preventing 'potential or actual dependency problems' which lie within her area of competence in order to satisfy her client's fundamental needs. Six main actual or potential problems were identified with which Jamie and his mother required nursing intervention (Fig. 9.2). Parents are encouraged to participate in their child's care as much as they are able, and can perform a number of activities (Sacharin, 1980), such as bathing, feeding and playing. Other potential problems were also recognised regarding Jamie's needs for keeping clean and dressed (including changing of nappies), safety and the availability of toys or games, but as these needs were normally met by Mrs T and she was to be resident with Jamie, they remained potential problems for the 'family unit'. Their consideration was required, however, in case Mrs T was unable to carry them out, as Jamie was not independent in satisfying these needs for himself.

Henderson (1966) advocates the setting of goals which may be long-term, intermediate or short-term, aimed at helping the patient regain independence in satisfying his fundamental needs. These goals may be based on problems identified during assessment, and on the presence of pathological states such as shock, respiratory distress or infection. Jamie's and Mrs T's problems were discussed with Mrs T and realistic short-term and

Fig. 9.1 Nursing assessment

Fundamental need	Normal	Present
Breathing	No problems.	Cold last 2–3 days. Barking cough started this evening; hoarse voice; noisy breathing; drawing in abdomen.
Eating and drinking	Three meals a day. Breakfast 7.00–8.00; lunch 12.00–12.30; supper 5.00 pm. Helps feed himself with spoon; manages food soft with 'lumps' – eats most foods – as family have. Drinks from teacher beaker, especially enjoys diluted orange juice.	Off food but drinking well until this evening – easily starts coughing and gets tired if drinking.
Elimination	Wears nappies day and night. Sits on potty after lunch for 10–15 mins. Not yet fully toilet trained.	No difference noticed today.
Mobilisation	Walking for last six weeks but needs supervision – falls often but gets up again.	Still walking as usual.
Sleep/rest	Usually has a nap after lunch for one hour. Goes to bed after bath – 6.00–6.30. Sleeps well through the night. Has 'cuddly blanket' to hold in bed.	Slight cough last night. Unable to settle this evening. Very restless; starts coughing when lying down.
Dressing/clothes	Helps dress himself – mostly done by parents.	No changes.
Temperature	No central heating in house which is near stream so tends to be damp at times. No problems normally with body temperature.	Slight pyrexia on admission; looks flushed and feels hot.
Washing/hair/skin	Bathed most evenings before bed. No problems normally.	Skin good, no nappy rash. Few small old bruises on legs and knees from falling over.
Safety/environment	Allowed to explore but parents aware of need for supervision at home. Puts toys in his mouth.	No changes.
Communication	No problems with hearing or sight. Saying some words and continually 'babbling'. Understands commands from parents e.g. 'Give it to mummy', 'Come to daddy'.	Not really talking. Clinging to mother. Mother very worried – has never seen him like this before.
Worship	Has been christened but parents not regular church goers.	
Work/occupation	Parents are self-employed and work from home. Jamie looked after part of the day by a child-minder – Lizzie (in his own home).	Jamie 'disturbing' normal schedule.
Play/recreation	Very aware of colours, shapes, etc. Builds a tower to two bricks.	Lost interest – very quickly losing concentration.
Learning/discovery	Always exploring. Inquisitive about things.	Lost interest this evening.

Fig. 9.2 Problem identification

Problems identified (A = actual, P = potential)	Nursing aim/goal
1 A Difficulty in breathing normally.	(a) Jamie will be able to breathe more easily within four hours. Shown by decreased breathing noise and less restlessness. (b) Jamie will be able to breathe normally.
2 A Difficulty in taking fluids due to cough/tiredness.	Jamie will have an adequate oral fluid intake (at least 750–1000 ml in 24 hours).
3 A Jamie is not having sufficient rest for his needs.	Jamie will not become over-tired or distressed and will have sufficient rest for his needs as demonstrated by a return to normal sleep pattern.
4 A Pyrexial on admission. Presence of infection may affect Jamie's ability to control his temperature.	Jamie's axillary temperature will not exceed 37.9°C.
5 A Jamie not communicating as normal. P Staff may be less aware of his needs than his mother.	Jamie's and mother's needs for communication will be met. Mrs T will express satisfaction at this.
6 A Mrs T has never seen a child with croup before and is not aware of the necessary care and observation.	Mrs T will learn how to look after Jamie when he has croup and how to provide humidity. She will express her confidence in providing this.

intermediate patient-centred goals were then set (Fig. 9.2). Observable results were identified by which evaluation of their progress and the success of nursing actions could take place.

A written care plan should be drawn up and modified according to the outcomes from nursing action (Henderson, 1972). She recommends that the plan of care should take into account the patient's normal habits so that the daily routine is changed as little as possible. Much of this was made possible for Jamie because his mother was providing the majority of his basic care.

Henderson is not explicit in recommending particular interventions, but Adam (1980) suggests that modes such as reinforcing, substituting and completing are used. Henderson (1966) does, however, advocate nursing taking place alongside medical intervention, so medical treatments which involve nursing action (such as use of drug therapy) also require documentation.

Chinn and Jacobs (1983) demonstrate that Henderson believes there is always a role for the family in health care, but again she is not explicit about the way this should be carried out. As already stated, therefore, Watson's (1983) recommendations about the family unit were incorporated into the way care was planned (Fig. 9.3).

For Jamie, nursing action entailed supporting Mrs T in caring for him and carrying out the activities she felt unable to do or lacked sufficient knowledge to do. These included observing Jamie, recording his pulse and respirations and providing humidity. As he progressed, however, and Mrs T gained more confidence, she gradually took a more active role in these interventions and was taught by nursing staff the principles of humidity and the complications to observe for whilst Jamie was breathing.

In order to evaluate the effectiveness of care using Henderson's (1966) model, the extent to which the goals set at the planning stage have been met should be determined, and the fundamental needs or problems identified at assessment as requiring nursing intervention should also be examined. Evaluation is not necessarily an end stage however, but may also entail a reassessment of needs and subsequent alterations of goals and nursing actions (Wright, 1985). On the other hand,

Fig. 9.3   Nursing action

1A	(a)	Mother present to help calm Jamie. Humidity provided (by croupette or vaporiser) to prevent airways swelling or drying up. Close observation as for problem 3.
	(b)	Keep Jamie calm and prevent complications by reporting any deterioration promptly. Educate Mrs T in the use of humidity.
2A		Offer small drinks often when awake – enjoys diluted orange juice from a teacher beaker. Record intake and output and total daily at midnight. Inform medical staff if total below 750 ml in 24 hours. Provide for food that he likes in case he wishes to eat.
3A		Close observation (without disturbing Jamie) of colour, type of breathing, recession of chest or for increasing restlessness or agitation. Report presence of any of the above problems, especially if combined with rising pulse and respiratory rates. Observe and record pulse and respirations every half-hour until improvement noticed, then record hourly overnight. If no improvement within 2 hours, inform medical staff. Raise head of bed by lifting mattress – no pillows. Ensure he has his cuddly blanket to hold in bed. Allow Jamie to rest after lunch, and settle to bed about 6 pm as usual.
4P	(a)	Ensure Jamie is appropriately dressed in cool clothes. To wear minimum clothing if feeling hot. Keep room cool especially if Jamie feels very warm.
	(b)	Record his axillary temperature every 2 hours, taking care not to disturb his sleep if possible.
	(c)	Paracetamol elixir is prescribed and may be given at not less than 4-hourly intervals if his temperature exceeds 37.5°C.
5A/P		Mother resident with Jamie – their nurse to ensure:
	(a)	opportunities given to discuss Jamie's care and management;
	(b)	mother encouraged to give as much of Jamie's care as she feels able;
	(c)	mother has sufficient rest;
	(d)	Mr T, Samuel, Lizzie and others encouraged to visit or phone.
6A		Ensure Mrs T has plenty of opportunities to learn about croup and humidity and how to recognise any complications that may arise.

a discharge evaluation may be made when fundamental needs are satisfied without nursing intervention and the patient goes home (Fig. 9.4).

For Jamie, the goals identified at the planning stage were met quickly and Mrs T rapidly gained confidence in caring for him, particularly in learning how to recognise croup and how to prevent Jamie from becoming too breathless. She could also identify occasions when she would need to call for assistance from her general practitioner. Within two days the family had become fully independent in satisfying Jamie's fundamental needs, so nursing intervention was no longer required.

Drug therapy

As croup is usually a viral illness, O'Dwyer (1985) and Barrell and Barnes (1985) argue that antibiotics are of little benefit and should therefore not be prescribed. However Coles (1977) does advocate the use of ampicillin because he considers it will decrease the incidence of secondary bacterial infection. O'Dwyer admits there may be occasions when a doctor feels 'obliged' to prescribe an antibiotic. The values which underline such an obligation may take their origins from the medical model which favours physical interventions.

The literature also demonstrates uncertainty about the use of sedation. O'Dwyer (1985) does not recommend its use as it may depress respirations or may mask the restlessness associated with hypoxia. Coles (1977), whilst acknowledging that heavy sedation may produce these effects, nevertheless believes that light sedation may help by allaying fears caused by hospital admission.

The only drug therapy prescribed for Jamie was paracetamol for its antipyretic effect, and only two doses were required throughout his stay. Sedation is not used for children with croup in the unit, and antibiotics are only prescribed if the child has started a course of treatment prior to admission.

Evaluation of the model in use

Wright (1986) believes that a nursing model should not be imposed but should allow nurses to explore

Fig. 9.4 Evaluation

Review date or time	Evaluation	Date
1 (a) 19.7 Within 4 hours – 01.30 hours	Has settled to sleep and breathing less noisily – **goal met**.	19.7
(b) Ongoing	Jamie now breathing more normally.	20.7
2 Ongoing Daily	24.00, 18.7. Small drinks taken regularly overnight. 24.00, 19.7. About 900 ml taken in 24 hours – **goal met**.	20.7

3 In 2 hours
    18.7 23.00 hours
    Ongoing
	Less recession, pulse and respiratory rates settling – **improvement**.
	Jamie has not become over-tired or distressed and has had sufficient rest for his needs.
		20.7

4 (a) Ongoing
    (b) 2-hourly
    (c) 4-hourly
	19.7. Temperature 37.9°C at 18.00 hours.
	Paracetamol given with effect – temperature 36.6°C at 20.00 hours. Temperature has since remained below 37.5°C – **problem resolved**.
		20.7

5 Ongoing	Mrs T says their needs for communication have been met satisfactorily throughout their stay.	20.7
6 Ongoing	Mrs T now expresses confidence in coping with Jamie when he has croup and feels able to recognise when she needs further help.	20.7

their practice rather than restricting it. He also warns that models focusing on the patient alone with insufficient consideration of the nurses or the social setting are of little benefit. Henderson's model of nursing (1966) is now familiar to many nurses and has been used as a framework for the documentation of care in this health district and others for some time. The model has been applied in a number of different settings and Aggleton and Chalmers (1985) believe this may indicate that Henderson's approach is closer to an overall theory of nursing than many others.

Henderson (1972) points out that special nursing problems may be posed by age, emotional state, social status, culture and intellect as well as nutritional and physiological conditions. All these variables may affect a person's ability to satisfy their fundamental needs. This chapter has attempted to consider the use of Henderson's model (1966) as a framework for managing the care of children, thus the special problems posed by age are particularly relevant. Most published examples of Henderson's model study its use in caring for adults with mainly physiological problems, however, and the documentation used within the health district in which Jamie was nursed was devised for general use, so the special needs of children are not always

considered. New documentation has therefore been designed for use in the paediatric unit using this model and has been applied here.

To successfully meet the special needs of children consideration of more than just their immediate problems is essential, according to Watson (1983). Care should include providing opportunities for play and education and in particular, should allow parents to be included in their child's care as appropriate (Belson, 1985). Buchanan (1983) makes the pertinent point that children are not small adults, but are individuals who are developing physically, psychologically, socially and educationally whether ill or not. Problems may be created, due to the effects of hospitalisation on a developing child if these special needs are ignored. When caring for sick children, therefore, Buchanan argues that the nurse's role must include that of communicator – with the doctor, child and parents; of educator – in teaching families how to cope with their child's illness whether temporary or long term; and of facilitator to recognise the need for other support as necessary. Miles (1985) even alerts us to the fact that in some cases a parent's need for care may be as great or greater than the child's.

All the above factors can be taken into account

when using Henderson's model of nursing as a framework for care, since she stresses (1972) the importance of an 'interpreter/communicator role' and believes a nurse is 'obliged to teach', whether consciously or not. In addition, as already stated, she advocates a team approach to care, the nurse working with other health carers, all of whom have a greater or lesser role to play in individualised care leading to the re-establishment of the patient's or family's independence.

Although Henderson does not specifically advocate use of the nursing process, she does emphasise (1966, 1972) the importance of an analytical and empathetic approach to managing care. The four stages of the nursing process – i.e. assessment, planning, implementation and evaluation – as described by Kratz (1979) are all included in Henderson's model of nursing, and she outlines (1982) a number of advantages of using the process. She continues however, that it 'ignores the subjective or intuitive aspect of nursing and the role of experience, logic and expert opinion'. This contradicts much that is written about the nursing process, for example Yura and Walsh (1978) who argue that it should be 'organised, systematic and deliberate' thus suggesting a move away from the traditional, intuitive foundation upon which nursing was practised. In addition, Aggleton and Chalmers (1984) point out that the nursing process provides nurses with a basic plan from which any model may be implemented, and that nursing models themselves are logically developed from a body of knowledge and understanding that aims to make nursing practice more informed and less intuitive.

Henderson's list of fourteen fundamental needs provides an effective basis for assessing an individual's, and a family's, needs. Henderson (1972) believes that all fourteen needs are equal in importance. Care must be taken during assessment that those needs considered first do not assume greater significance. Fitzpatrick and Whall (1983) believe Henderson's definition of nursing has the potential to be sensitive to the whole person, but the physiological aspects receive greater emphasis. Adam (1980) however considers that each fundamental need has psychological, social and cultural dimensions, and Henderson herself (1972)

describes more than just physiological aspects of each.

Henderson (1972) accepts the constraints of achieving complete independence for a child, due to its age, but although acknowledging a role for the family in planning and implementing care, she is inexplicit about the form it should take. This contrasts with Orem's model of nursing (1980) which describes a clear role for parents, calling them dependent care agents. As previously described, however, Watson's (1983) suggestions that the family unit be considered rather than the child in isolation have been successfully implemented, thus increasing the contribution of Henderson's model in managing the care of children.

The importance of development as an ongoing process has already been stressed by Buchanan (1983) and is a vital factor to be considered when planning and implementing care for children. Again, Henderson is imprecise about developmental needs but physical, emotional, social and educational aspects can all be assessed using Henderson's model of nursing. For a child requiring short-term care or who is very young (for instance pre-school), these aspects are closely linked and it may be difficult to separate them, but for an older child who has started school, who may require longer-term care, each aspect must be given careful consideration. In these circumstances, needs relating to physical development may be included with mobility, dressing, washing and playing; social and emotional development can be considered with communication and play/recreational needs, and educational development can be explored together with working and learning, discovering and satisfying curiosity. Assessing developmental needs may prove difficult for some nurses. However this should pose few problems for those with sick children's or nursery nurse training, or those with considerable experience who have acquired the skills.

Difficulties may arise, however, when caring for adolescents, since sexuality is important in their development but is not mentioned by Henderson, although Adam (1980) includes this aspect within communication needs.

To summarise, the use of Henderson's model appears to be successful in managing the care of children, due to her stress on individualised care and her inclusion of all members of the team in delivering care. Involvement of the family and consideration of developmental needs, although not clearly defined by Henderson, are both factors to which she makes reference in describing her model of nursing, and these may make a useful contribution to care. With training and experience in the field of paediatric nursing, the model can be appropriately interpreted, thereby extending its contribution to the management of the care of children.

References

Adam E 1980 *To be a Nurse.* WB Saunders, Toronto.

Aggleton P & Chalmers H 1984 Defining the terms. *Nursing Times*, September 5: 24–28.

Aggleton P & Chalmers H 1984 Henderson's model. *Nursing Times*, March 6: 33–35.

Barrell E & Barnes G 1985 Croup: To treat or not to treat. *Nursing Times*, August 21: 41–43.

Belson P 1985 Children are special. *Nursing Times*, October 16: 34.

Bowlby J 1951 *Maternal Care & Mental Health.* WHO, Geneva.

Brunner LS & Suddarth DS 1986 *The Lippincott Manual of Paediatric Nursing*, 2nd ed. Harper & Row, London.

Buchanan M 1983 The Sick Child. *Nursing Times*, February 23: 66–69.

Burr S 1984 Children's rights – and wrongs. *Nursing Times*, November 21: 16–18.

Chinn PL & Jacobs MK 1983 *Theory and Nursing: A Systematic Approach.* CV Mosby, St Louis.

Coles HMT 1977 Croup. *Nursing Times*, October 20: 1634–1635.

Drinkwater C 1984 Stridor in children. *Medicine in Practice*, February 1: 18–23.

Eichelberger KH, Kausman DH, Rundahl ME & Schwartz NE 1980 Self-care nursing plan: helping children to help themselves. *Pediatric Nursing*, 6, 3: 9–13.

Evans M 1985 Handled with care. *Nursing Times*, September 11: 32–36.

Fitzpatrick JJ & Whall AL (Eds) 1983 *Conceptual Models of Nursing: Analysis and Application.* Robert J Brady Co, Maryland.

Henderson V 1964 The nature of nursing. *American Journal of Nursing*, August: 62–68.

Henderson V 1966 *The Nature of Nursing: A Definition and its Implications, Practice, Research and Education.* Macmillan, New York.

Henderson V 1972 *Basic Principles of Nursing Care.* International Council of Nurses, Geneva.

Henderson V 1982 The nursing process: Is the title right? *Journal of Advanced Nursing*, 7, 2: 103–109.

Jolly J 1981 *The Other Side of Paediatrics.* Macmillan, London.

King H & David TJ 1982 *Applied Paediatric Nursing.* Pitman, London.

Kratz C 1979 *The Nursing Process.* Bailliere Tindall, London.

Maslow AH 1954 *Motivation and Personality.* Harper & Row, London.

Miles I 1985 A suitable case for treatment. *Nursing Times*, May 1: 48–50.

Milner AD 1984 Acute stridor in the pre-school child. *British Medical Journal*, 288: 811.

O'Dwyer P 1985 How I manage croup. *Pulse of Medicine*, June 8: 62.

Orem D 1980 *Nursing: Concepts of Practice.* McGraw-Hill, New York.

Platt H 1959 *Report of the Committee on the Welfare of Children in Hospital.* HMSO, London.

Roy C 1980 The Roy adaptation model. In *Conceptual Models for Nursing Practice*, JP Riehl & C Roy (Eds). Appleton-Century-Crofts, Norwalk.

Sacharin RM 1980 *Principles of Paediatric Nursing.* Churchill Livingstone, Edinburgh.

Thorndike EI 1940 *Human Nature and the Social Order.* Macmillan, New York.

Waechter EH & Blake FG 1976 *Nursing Care of Children*, 9th Ed. Lippincott, New York.

Watson R 1983 Paediatric care: Contrasts and developments. *Nursing Times*, December 21: 46–48.

Wright S 1985 Special assignment. *Nursing Times*, August 28: 36–37.

Wright S 1986 Developing and using a nursing model. In *Models for Nursing*, B Kershaw & J Salvage (Eds). John Wiley & Sons, Chichester.

Yura H & Walsh MB 1978 *The Nursing Process*, 3rd ed. Appleton-Century-Crofts, New York.

10

A way forward

Helen Chalmers

What have been presented in this book are eight care plans which describe and begin to evaluate seven models of nursing. A variety of care settings is in evidence and the patients concerned vary in age from the very young to the elderly. They share a need for nursing care which stemmed from problems within the cardiovascular or respiratory systems.

It is not the intention of this final chapter to restate what has gone before but rather to highlight a number of issues that seem pertinent to the continuing debate that needs to surround the use of nursing models.

Attitudes

Roy's Adaptation model (Roy, 1980) argues for careful consideration of the pooled effect of certain stimuli (focal, contextual and residual) on people's behaviour and their ability to adapt to the circumstances in which they find themselves. Residual stimuli are the values and beliefs held by individuals and may often be difficult to change. This should be regarded positively because values and beliefs are important in enabling us to make decisions that are consistent and with which we feel at ease. They form part of the attitudes we hold and their relative permanence has long interested psychologists.

In suggesting that nurses should look critically at the traditional ways in which nursing care has been planned and delivered, it should be remembered that most nurses will have valued and believed in whatever private image has guided the care they offer. It is to be expected therefore that some nurses will find the change of attitude demanded by certain nursing models difficult to adopt. Indeed this may serve as a safeguard against the uncritical acceptance of models or any other apparent innovation in nursing.

The study of care in Chapter 2 also serves to emphasise the effect of the residual stimuli of others on a person's ability to adapt. Here Lucy, a teenage girl with a medical diagnosis of asthma, was restricted in what she could do by the beliefs of others about the nature of asthma and the limitations it should impose on her. Such residual stimuli became contextual stimuli for Lucy.

Similarly if the beliefs of senior nurses are that models of nursing have nothing to offer and are best ignored or discussed in isolated classrooms in schools or colleges of nursing, this then will hamper the critical evaluation of models by those nurses who wish to explore their potential usefulness. The residual stimuli of one group of nurses might then be the contextual or focal stimuli of another group.

Sharing of knowledge

A number of the care plans presented have in some way discussed the importance of the sharing of knowledge with others as a means of offering those people some control over the situation in which they find themselves. Chapter 4 is one such example. Perhaps a way forward in the continuing evaluation of nursing models is for nurses to share their experiences of what models might offer with each other and with other health carers and patients.

The use of nursing models, moreover, might facilitate the sharing of knowledge between nurses. If traditionally nurses have planned and delivered care on the basis of the medical model and their own past nursing experiences, their private image has been, in part, unique to them. Such a situation does not lend itself to the dissemination of knowledge in a systematic and coherent way. It may mean that certain expertise within nursing rests with individuals and is rarely or incompletely shared. Were care to be organised around a nursing model it might be possible to discuss more effectively and learn from the experience of others.

Accountability

> Each registered nurse, midwife and health visitor is accountable for his or her practice ...
> (UKCC 1984)

Central to the notion of accountability is the ability of each registered nurse, midwife or health visitor to justify the ways in which he or she practises. The use of a nursing model with the nursing process should enable such justifications to be made.

However, as has been evident throughout this book, most nursing models have room for further development and there is a wealth of nursing literature, not specifically model based, which can also be used to provide rationales for nursing interventions.

It is likely that the central premises of a model will indicate the kind of nursing and other literature that might be useful in helping nurses to account for the helping strategies they adopt.

Thus a model with an emphasis on the development of a relationship between nurse and patient should be enhanced by reference to the extensive literature on communication and rapport building. A model that encourages independence or self-care might be implemented more successfully if used in conjunction with literature about helping individuals develop physical skills and feelings of self-worth. A nurse wishing to work with a model that recognises the importance to individuals of the roles they can adopt within a given situation, may find the model easier to implement following an exploration of the sociological and psychological literature concerning role theories.

Three issues have been selected for further consideration in this last chapter, namely the importance of attitudes, the sharing of knowledge, and accountability. Hopefully readers of this book will find many other ideas of sufficient interest to encourage them to take up the challenges offered by the introduction of nursing models.

What has been presented here is necessarily limited in what it can contribute to the essential evaluation of the usefulness of nursing models in practice. What it can do is value the work of individual nurses, many of whom work in less than ideal clinical settings but who nevertheless have been able to use a nursing model, attempt to evaluate its role in improving the quality of care, and share their conclusions with others.

References

Roy C 1980 The Roy adaptation model. In *Conceptual Models for Nursing Practice*, JP Riehl & C Roy (Eds). Appleton-Century-Crofts, Norwalk.
UKCC 1984 *Code of Professional Conduct*, 2nd ed. UKCC, London.

Index